Healthy Mind

First published by Busybird Publishing 2015
Copyright © 2015 Busybird Publishing

ISBN 978-1-925260-78-6

Busybird Publishing has asserted their right under the Copyright, Designs and Patents Act 1988 to be identified as the author of this work. The information in this book is based on the author's experiences and opinions. The publisher specifically disclaims responsibility for any adverse consequences, which may result from use of the information contained herein. Permission to use information has been sought by the author. Any breaches will be rectified in further editions of the book.

All rights reserved. No part of this publication may be reproduced, stored in or introduced into a retrieval system, or transmitted in any form, or by any means (electronic, mechanical, photocopying, recording or otherwise) without the prior written permission of the author. Any person who does any unauthorised act in relation to this publication may be liable to criminal prosecution and civil claims for damages. Enquiries should be made through the publisher.

Cover image: Kev Howlett, Busybird Publishing
Cover design: Busybird Publishing
Layout and typesetting: Busybird Publishing

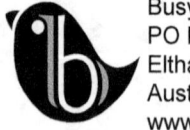

Busybird Publishing
PO Box 855
Eltham Victoria
Australia 3095
www.busybird.com.au

'If you correct your mind, the rest of your life will fall into place.'

– Lao Tzu

Contents

Foreword *Tim Ferguson*	i
Behind a Healthy Mind *Sara Van Hecke*	1
The Sounds of Resonance *Anthony Kilner*	13
The Written Word as Therapy *Blaise van Hecke*	35
Creating and Maintaining a Healthy Mind *Dr Talia Steed*	51
The Benefits of Kinesiology *Debbie Rossi*	65
Sacred Harmony *Mary Jo Mc Veigh*	81
Challenging Your Mind for Greatness *Samantha Jansen*	101
The Art of a Healthy Mind *Isolde Martin*	119
Trust and Respect *Galen Dean Loven*	131
Write For Your Life *Les Zigomanis*	151
Biographies	169

comedian

Foreword

Tim Ferguson

The mind works in mysterious ways. It is the largest, most complex computing system in the known universe. The mind is creative, destructive, capable of great works and terrible crimes. The mind is its own greatest enemy and strongest ally. So what do you do when your mind turns upon itself? The wizardry of psychiatry and the cold motive processes of meditation, yoga or physical exercise are useful against the onslaught of your own mind against your will.

Yet the best defensive weapon against a dysfunctional or destructive mental state is your own mental resilience.

I have multiple sclerosis. It's a new logical condition that erodes the protective layers of the nerves in my brain and spine. The effects of this erosion can range from numbness, neurological pain, pins and needles, vision impairment, slurred speech, brain fog, problems with mobility and agility, numbness and involuntary muscular spasms. Crazy, unpredictable stuff. The condition is different for every patient, manifesting in its own smorgasbord of wackiness.

Whatever the manifestations of MS may be, the most reliable ways to maintain a useful and productive life are simple.

Positivity and willpower are the most readily

available tools for fighting the darker moods that frustrations bring.

Using optimism and a little stubbornness, I have managed to work around the world in the stressful and challenging entertainment industries, making television shows, live comedy shows, books and feature films. It's an existence fraught with conflict, pressure and risk. No drug or treatment can work as reliably as positive thinking. This sounds trite, I know, but there is no other known behaviour that can reliably achieve resilience.

Everyone feels pressures in their life. Whatever those pressures may be, it is worth devoting a little time each day to refreshing our awareness of the things we love, the people who love us, our dreams and how we hope to achieve them. We must enjoy our journeys even if we know our destinations will forever elude us. What else are we going to do?

This book has some innovative and simple suggestions for maintaining a positive outlook, avoiding common behavioural and cognitive tricks, learning to endure the fickleness of our abilities and generating new approaches to dealing with the problems that can plague our minds.

This is a rare and important book. None of us completely knows our own mind. But this book can help us all explore our minds and the way they function.

Here is your chance to embrace the mystery.

Tim Ferguson

psychologist

Behind a Healthy Mind

Sara Van Hecke

What is a healthy mind from a psychologist's perspective?

Is it about 'sanity' and, if so, how do we define sanity? Isn't this largely a social and cultural construction? Is a healthy mind about having clarity? Or is it about happiness? Is it about the absence of a mental disorder as defined by our diagnostic manuals? Is it about level of functioning?

The questions are endless and the answers diverse!

Psychologists are trained to consider the etiology of any patient's symptoms in order to formulate treatment. Our view of cause and subsequent treatment can, in part, depend on the psychologist's approach.

I posed the question of how to define a healthy mind to some colleagues. I thought the answer would be somewhat uniform. After all, we are scientists, working in an evidence-based way. To my surprise, there were minimal commonalities in the answers. The responses, in large, depended on the approach of the psychologist.

According to a psychologist practising positive psychology, a healthy mind is about flourishing – about a person functioning at their potential. Someone with a healthy mind, from this perspective, would have the resilience to cope with life's challenges, would relate well to others, would feel that life is meaningful and would lead a creative and productive life. Perhaps this suggests that someone with an unhealthy mind would focus on the negative rather than the positive, interpreting daily stressors as more stressful than others might find them.

In this sense, the positive psychologist has some overlap with the cognitive behavioural psychologist/therapist. Cognitive Behaviour Therapy (CBT) posits that someone with an unhealthy mind has unhealthy thinking habits, like focusing on the negative all the time, or 'black and white' thinking, whereby a person views situations as 'all' bad, or 'all' their fault, and cannot bring a balanced perspective to situations. The result of these unhealthy thinking habits is that we feel bad. Therapy focuses on changing our thinking habits in order to change how we feel.

CBT, in turn, has some overlap with Mindfulness Based Cognitive Therapy (MBCT). MBCT, like CBT, posits that our thoughts have the ability to wreak havoc on us. We can have several people experiencing the same event but each will feel differently about that event depending on how we think about it.

The difference between CBT and MBCT is that MBCT doesn't assume that your thoughts are irrational or wrong, just that they aren't so useful. The MBCT therapist uses mindfulness and meditation to teach their client to not buy into these thoughts so much. To instead be able to respond to triggers with awareness, acceptance and without judgement. The unhealthy mind here is really the reactive, unaware, judgemental mind.

The psychoanalyst believes that unconscious forces from our past are impacting on our current functioning. Our personality consists of three elements: the Id, the Ego and the Superego. The Id is the impulsive part, the part driven by pleasure – *I want what I want and I want it now!* The Superego is the disciplinarian, the moral compass. The Superego uses guilt to try to temper our Id. The Ego tries to balance the two. In doing so, it is trying to protect the person from stress. Too much Superego and we would crumble with the weight of guilt; too much Id and we would struggle in the real world. The Ego tries to protect the person from struggle with uncomfortable feelings and if necessary employs 'defences' to prevent unconscious thoughts from becoming conscious. From this perspective, the unhealthy mind is a highly defended one.

There were more approaches and many stimulating discussions with colleagues about their opinions in relation to this topic. What became apparent through these discussions is that there are no purists. That is, nobody approached their work using a pure form of any of these theories at the expense of other theories. It seemed that all psychologists have one main approach that underpins their conceptualisation of their client, but they draw on other approaches to help broaden their thinking about their client.

The longer I do this work, the more aware I become of what and how much I DON'T know. This is a good sign, my supervisor told me. It seems to me that to wed yourself to one approach over any other doesn't allow you to bring an openness to your client. Instead, a strict adherence to one psychological theory suggests that you are trying to fit your client into a preconceived notion of what is wrong with them and why. Humans are too diverse for this and the world too complex.

So back to my thoughts about what constitutes a healthy mind. That definition would differ from client to client and would largely come from their own descriptions of their suffering.

Added to that, I'm drawing on theories to check whether any of them make sense with what the client is reporting but also I'm looking for clues from the client about what they are up for, e.g. being challenged on their defences or practicing some mindfulness.

I'm drawing on my experience about what works with what and then I'm weaving in all the information that I'm gleaning from our dynamic animated conversations: where are they in their life; what was their childhood like; what has worked for them; what hasn't; what is their personality like; are they more left brained, right brained; do they exercise; how do they eat; what are their strengths; their vulnerabilities; how resourced are they (in all sorts of ways); and what are their relationships like. On and on it goes, building the relationship, getting to know them. It's a collaboration, it's an exploration.

When you ask your client, 'What is it you want from this process?', these are some of the answers:

- 'I want to be happier'
- 'I want to be more creative'
- 'I want to feel more grounded'

- 'I want to be calmer'
- 'I want my relationship to be happier, more grounded or calmer'.

It's rarely, 'I want more money' or 'I want a bigger house'. When clients elaborate, they tell me things like, 'I'm just so busy', 'I never have any time', 'it's hard to switch off', 'there's no time for me', or 'I'm not very good at doing nothing'. But perhaps the most often-cited reason for coming to see a psychologist is loneliness. Clients feel lonely, disconnected, isolated.

It seems difficult to imagine that loneliness is so prevalent in today's world. Modern technology means that we are always connected. But this connection via our mobile phones, computers and the internet appears to be contributing to the inability of people to form meaningful connections.

More than half of all British teenagers spend around thirty hours per week using technology other than that used in school, with the majority of that time spent on social media. So shouldn't we feel more connected, less isolated?

Social researchers are finding that those teenagers who are struggling with depression, or are socially anxious, shy or who do not have good social skills are more likely to develop compulsive internet usage, while those less anxious and more extroverted are out there engaging in healthy social activities. These healthy activities include playing sport, being involved in extracurricular activities and just simply hanging out with friends.

As therapists treating depressed, lonely people, treating the depression is only part of the issue. Helping the client make friends is likely to be the more valuable part of treatment. Research has shown that if we were limited to only offering one thing to our depressed clients out of antidepressants, talking therapy, exercise and/or good diet, ECT, sleep hygiene, or social support, the social support is going to offer the most impact over anything else.

So I worry in this sense about the future. If social media and phone usage are replacing more meaningful social contact, what does this mean for our social connectedness? How, in turn, will technology affect the evolution of our brains and, in turn, our minds?

Our ability to access information instantly means that we are experiencing the input of information at greater levels than ever before, but this does not mean that we are able to digest this information at any meaningful level. While the brain does appear to have infinite capacity, there appears to be evidence that we are using our brain differently because of our relationship with technology.

Remember the time when you would meet friends in the city and have to co-ordinate times and places and think about which tram you would catch and have contingency plans if you lost one another? None of that is necessary anymore; you just make some vague plan and ring or text them when you are close. So what happens to the planning parts of our brain, or the ability to focus attention, or our memory, if information is coming at us as such?

Already, clients come in saying that they are engaging in 'checking' behaviours around social media and their phone. Some are reporting that they wake frequently during the night to check Facebook. It is so bad for some that they feel distressed by it, and are unable to function as they would like to. It's given birth to a new breed of unhealthy minds.

Finally, it's impossible to talk about what constitutes a healthy mind without referring to self-care – in particular the impact of lifestyle on how we feel. It seems like common sense that if we feel better physically we are likely to feel better emotionally. But it's not just common sense; it has been researched and there is no disputing that how we treat our body impacts on the health of our mind.

In my own work, I am interested in some basics: Sleep, Diet, Exercise and Relationships.

All of us have experienced a worsened mood after a bad night's sleep, and studies have shown that sleep deprivation has a significant effect on our mood. For example, studies have shown that people who have been diagnosed with insomnia are five times more likely to develop major depression and twenty times more likely to develop panic disorder. Furthermore, not only does sleep quality affect mood but mood also affects sleep quality.

Anxiety and stress make us more agitated, making it harder to settle at night, leading to poor sleep and greater anxiety as a result. Looking at good sleep hygiene can go a long way to improving client's presenting symptoms and will always be a basic part of assessment when a new client walks in the door.

We tend to know that our mood can impact on what we choose to eat (i.e. the impact of mood on food). How many times have we felt a bit low and reached for chocolate or other goodies only to regret it later? There has been a growing interest of late about how food intake can impact on how we feel, i.e. the effect on food on mood, a field that is becoming known as *Nutritional Neuroscience*.

Brain chemicals such as serotonin, norepinephrine and dopamine affect the way we feel. Food intake plays a big part in maintaining optimal levels of these chemicals in the brain. Around the world, research is showing links between diet and mood. Lower dietary intake of foliate, zinc, essential fatty acids and vitamins B1, B2 and C are linked to higher rates of depression.

Research into Omega-3 has shown that lower levels of Omega-3 are linked to lower levels of serotonin and dopamine. Japan has shown to have lower rates of depression than those consuming a regular Western diet. A strong hypothesis for this is that Japanese people consume more fish, fish being a great source of essential fatty acids. A study in the UK backs this. It showed that people in the UK who consumed more essential fatty acids as measured by their seafood intake had lower rates of depression, post-natal depression, seasonal affective disorder and bipolar affective disorder. Other studies have shown that when people diagnosed with depression take Omega-3 supplements, their symptoms improve.

Scientists think that both Omega-3 and

Omega-6 need to be consumed in equal parts. Omega-6 signals the immune system to turn on while Omega-3 signals the immune system to turn off. We tend to hear about the need to keep our Omega-3 levels up more because Western diets tend to be deficient in Omega-3. However, while taking an Omega-3 supplement has shown to help with depressive symptoms, taking too much has shown no improvement in symptoms.

This is such a small sample of the research connecting nutrition to brain health. The research in this area is growing and many psychologists today would assess lifestyle issues as part of their assessment of their client. Subsequently, many psychologists might make recommendations to their clients about improving diet as part of their overall treatment plan.

Exercise impacts mood in a number of ways. Many people who are stressed will report feeling better just five minutes into some exercise, while research has shown that those who engage in some moderate exercise three to four times a week are more likely to show improvements in depressive symptoms than those who don't. Researchers don't know exactly how exercise promotes these types of benefits, but one theory is that exercise helps release more serotonin in the brain. Serotonin is the neurotransmitter targeted by some antidepressant medications. Another theory is simply that exercise helps regulate sleep. Exercise is also thought to make us more confident and less likely to get anxious about a variety of stressors.

Relationships, too, matter in a variety of ways.

When we are struggling with thoughts that are impacting on our mood, it helps to have people that we feel close enough to, to talk to about these thoughts. Getting another perspective often helps us to stop the ruminating and hence, feel better.

Having relationships with people also helps us to not feel the discomfort of loneliness. Loneliness often includes feelings of sadness or anxiety about not belonging or being part of a community. Humans are social beings and tend to survive better in groups, hence the instinct towards meaningful relationships with others.

So, in summary, defining a 'healthy mind' will vary from person to person and perhaps from clinician to clinician. However, there is no doubting that in treating an unhealthy mind, no matter what the suffering, I have my basic checklist:

1. Quality of Sleep: if you are fatigued, everything will be harder.
2. Diet: good nutrition makes us feel more vital and helps your brain to fire more efficiently.
3. Exercise: we don't know how, but research has shown again and again, that exercise improves mood.
4. Relationships: having good friends and family gives us a sense of belonging and makes us feel more supported when life gets a little tougher.

psychic medium

The Sounds of Resonance
Anthony Kilner

Vibrational healing has existed in our world from the very beginning of time. Through the uplifting melody of musical instruments, the soothing human voice, or the relaxing sounds of nature, we have all experienced some therapeutic benefit from vibration and sound. As soon as we are conceived and enfolded within our mother's womb, we are soothed by her voice. That voice, the vibration of sound and love, resonates through to our tiny, developing bodies. This is vibrational healing at its core.

I should say at the outset that I am not comfortable with the term 'healing' or being called a 'healer'. I prefer 'energy worker' or 'energy facilitator', as that's essentially what I do – use energy, sound and vibration to help the body heal itself.

I also work on the principle that to help the body heal itself, a practitioner needs to work closely with their client to identify the core of their problem. Once that's done, the client can take the necessary steps to bring about their own self-healing.

Sound, music and vibration go hand in hand and, when coupled with colour, can be a powerful tool to help create a healthy mind and a healthy body. Before we head into the healing component of sound, it might help to understand a little of how we receive sound.

There are two ways we can feel and hear sound and vibration. The first is through our eardrums. Our eardrums pick up sound frequencies. The vibrations of those frequencies are then converted through our eardrums into a signal that our brain recognises as sound. In very basic terms we hear with our brains.

The second way we can feel vibration and sound is through our bodies. The average adult body is around sixty-five percent water, which is a great conductor for vibration and electrical signals. Sounds pass through our body, which signals our brains that we just felt and – on some level – *heard* something, even though it might be outside our normal hearing range.

Sound in technical terms is a longitudinal mechanical wave which creates a frequency. Frequency is measured by the number of cycles in the wave and is measured in Hertz (Hz). The frequency of the soundwave determines the pitch and tone of the sound. This is how we measure and rate our musical instruments, body parts and other sounds that surround us.

The average person can pick up on sounds that range from 20Hz to 20,000Hz. With age, this range can reduce markedly, all the way to full deafness, although even a deaf person can feel vibration and interpret what's happening around them. Many years ago I attended parties held by a deaf friend of mine. While the music was loud to those with normal hearing, the deaf people sat around with their feet on the floor and hands on the table picking up the beat and the rhythm of the music through the vibrations. It was an amazing experience, especially watching them move and groove to the music I could hear too loudly and they couldn't hear at all.

Animals, birds and the aquatic world pick up on sound frequencies and vibrations. Elephant hearing, for example, ranges from approximately 16Hz to 12,000Hz, while a bat varies from 2,000Hz to 110,000Hz. The humble goldfish runs from 20Hz to 3,000Hz, while dolphins communicate in the range of 20Hz to 150,000Hz, which is far superior to us mere humans. On the domestic side of things, dogs have a hearing range from 67Hz to 45,000Hz while cats have a brilliant range between 45Hz to 64,000Hz.

I'll be the first to admit I am not a scientist or a physicist or any sort of 'ologist' so for those inclined to do so, jump on the net and feel free to research the super tech details that are available if you are keen to know more about how sound works.

In my world, as a musician, medium and energy worker, I have experienced how sound can be used as a healing tool. Sounds move through our physical bodies, and our bodies on a cellular level react to the different frequencies of those sounds. Our bodies also reflect or refract sound, as do all objects. This reflection of sound can be used as a diagnostic tool, while the absorption of sound can be used to effect the healing itself.

On a diagnostic level, a single note (sound), such as that produced by a crystal singing bowl, will have a different resonance when it bounces back from different mediums such as wood, metal, liquid or the human body, due to the difference in density of the object. An energy worker can hear this difference in resonance as the crystal bowl is moved up and down alongside different organs in the body while the bowl is resonating. The sound reverberates through the body and comes back to us a bit like a radar so we can hear the variations in sound from different locations around the body. With practice and skill a practitioner can pick up on potential health problems from the sounds reverberating off the client's body.

The specific nature of what that problem might be would need to be investigated in detail and, not being a doctor, I would not make any sort of diagnosis.

On a healing level, all matter has its own natural frequency. Every particle in our body vibrates at a specific frequency, and when our body is unwell some of these frequencies can change or get out of sync. Vibrational healing introduces multiple frequencies to the body to excite change in the 'out-of-sync' vibrations. By using sound and vibration to get the body moving on a cellular level, the body will start to self-heal to the best of its ability.

There are other factors that contribute to the healing process, including regular exercise, the right nutrition, keeping the body well hydrated, and mental health.

There is also more to vibrational healing than just sound working on the physical body. Often people refer to the Mind, Body and Spirit, or Mind, Body and Soul. When it comes to vibrational healing, I refer to Mind, Body and Energy. It is important to analyse these three aspects of self and make sense of them in order to attain a healthy body, a healthy mind and create a happy life.

The **Body** is the complex flesh and blood component. It's the vehicle we use to get from birth to death. To achieve a healthy body we should be feeding it correctly, exercising it correctly, and giving it every chance to be the perfect vehicle to live in. If we consider the body down to a cellular level, it's made up of billions of cells, and has the ability to heal itself against disease and invasions. Genetically, the body holds the key to hereditary disease as well as external disease such as melanoma or asbestos. As we live out our lives and subject our body to the rigours of life, it reacts accordingly. From breaks, sprains and cancers to glowing health, the body, put simply, is amazing!

The **Mind** is a unique piece of the kit that works with and controls the body, taking its information from all the senses. Like a computer operating a vehicle, it uses every piece of external stimuli to allow us to react to any given situation. Like the *body*, the *mind* is unique. The mind makes sense of the reality around it and has the ability to reach into the spirit world, universe, or other dimensions, depending on your outlook on the world.

Our **Mind** is also amazing in that it allows us to achieve various states of consciousness. Our everyday consciousness is how we live and also make decisions and choices. The next level is our subconscious, which generally absorbs things our consciousness is too busy to notice. Then finally, our super consciousness, which connects us to our *higher self*, *Spirit* or *Soul* as some people might refer to it.

The third aspect of self to understand, even on a basic level, is the **Subtle Energy Body**. This is generated via the 'chakra' system, which creates our auric field. This electromagnetic energy field pulses and changes constantly and is unique to each person, like our DNA.

'Chakra' comes from Sanskrit and means 'wheel', 'turning', or 'wheel of light', and in Yogic circles the chakras are referred to as a vortex or whirlpool. While there are over 110 minor chakras around the body, most people reference the chakra system to the seven major chakras or the seven centres of spiritual power in the human body.

Each of the main chakras resonates at a specific frequency or hertz and these chakras are aligned with the endocrine system of the body. This means that our subtle body also works with the physical body and the mind to promote complete health and harmony on all levels.

Applying the same single note example on the body (previous page), the energetic body also responds to the sound and creates a resonance that can be heard. A practitioner must have a good understanding of both the physical and energetic bodies to help a client during a vibrational healing session.

The chakra frequencies also align to specific colours, which are transverse waves that can be matched in frequency to the hertz range. Colour and light are transverse waves of electromagnetic radiation which move from side to side, unlike sound which moves up and down. There is a spectrum of colour that is visible to the human eye and there are colours we can't see with the human eye, yet we know they exist, such as gamma rays or radio waves. In basic terms, this is why the use of colour during energy work complements the use of sound.

There is a raft of information in books and on the net about the chakras and how they work, although there seems to be some variations on which colour sits where within the Hertz scale. The details below are a summary I've put together from various sources that combines the elements of the major chakras to provide an insight as to how the different aspects of each chakra interact with the physical body.

Base Chakra (Red) Instincts/Fight or flight
Musical Note: C
Solfeggio Tone: UT – 396Hz
Chakra Frequency: 256Hz
Location: Perineal point between Anus and Genitals
Parts of the Body: Adrenal glands, Legs, Feet, Bones, Large Intestine, and Teeth

Sacral Chakra (Orange) Emotions
Musical Note: D
Solfeggio Tone: RE – 417Hz
Chakra Frequency: 288Hz
Location: Hypogastric Plexus; Genitals, Womb (just below the belly button)
Parts of the Body: Ovaries, Testicles, Womb, Genitals, Kidney, Bladder, and Circulatory System

Solar Plexus Chakra (Yellow) Mind/Mental Thoughts
Musical Note: E
Solfeggio Tone: MI – 528 Hz
Chakra Frequency: 320Hz
Location: Between the bottom of the sternum and the belly button
Parts of the Body: Pancreas, Adrenals, Digestive System, Muscles

Heart Chakra (Emerald Green) Compassion/Empathy
Musical Note: F
Solfeggio Tone: FA – 639Hz
Chakra Frequency: 341.3Hz
Location: Heart
Parts of the Body: Thymus, Lungs, Heart, Pericardium, Arms, Hands

Throat Chakra (Cobalt Blue) Communication
Musical Note: G
Solfeggio Tone: SOL – 741Hz
Chakra Frequency: 384Hz
Location: Throat
Parts of the Body: Thyroid, Parathyroid, Shoulders, Neck, Arms, Hands

Third Eye Chakra (Indigo) Intuition
Musical Note: A
Solfeggio Tone: LA – 852Hz – Returning to Spiritual Order
Chakra Frequency: 426.7Hz
Location: The point between the eyebrows
Parts of the Body: Pineal, Eyes

Crown Chakra (Violet White) Cosmic Awareness
Musical Note: B
Solfeggio Tone: TI – 963 Hz – Solfeggio Higher Frequency
Chakra Frequency: 480Hz
Location: Top of the head
Parts of the Body: Pituitary Gland, Central Nervous System, Cerebral Cortex

When looking at our bodies as a whole like this and understanding that mind, body and energy all interact and react with each other, it becomes easier to see why using music and sound in our everyday lives is so important to promote a balanced healthy body.

By controlling the sounds we hear through music or singular sounds or tones, we can change the way our physical bodies respond. For example, low frequency sound waves can drain energy from the body while high frequency sound waves excite and draw energy into the body.

The more excited our bodies become, the more energy we can use. This is why dancing and music is exhilarating and exhausting and leave the mind in a happy state of being.

Alternatively, working around an engine that drones on and on, can actually drain us of energy, leaving us feeling flat.

People don't need to be rocket scientists or doctors to understand how sound, vibration, and colour all work together on our physical, mental and energetic bodies.

In everyday life, just listening to music, playing

instruments or even listening to the sounds of nature, can have an incredibly positive impact on our mental and physical health and wellbeing.

Meditation and Vibrational Healing at Home

One of the best ways I know to achieve a positive result with vibrational healing at home is to do it in conjunction with meditation or in a deep, relaxed state.

Having said that, I often hear from people that they can't meditate or that they have tried to meditate and nothing happened other than they kept thinking about stuff. This is the most common problem that crops up – the conscious mind chatters too much!

Jon Kabat-Zinn, founder of the Mindfulness-Based Stress Reduction program at the University of Massachusetts Medical Centre, says, 'Mindfulness means paying attention in a particular way, on purpose, in the present moment, and nonjudgmentally.' I find this to be a very succinct way of putting it.

While studying in India with Tibetan monks, I sat in on a lengthy discussion on what the monks call 'Monkey Mind' and 'Mindfulness Meditation'. This lecture – which went on for more than three hours – was all about using all the sounds occurring around you and allowing yourself permission to relax and therefore meditate with purpose to be at peace with oneself.

I found this lecture absolutely fascinating and there was plenty of time to practice what was being discussed. We meditated to classical music, Tibetan music, traffic noises, and even everyday noises such as dogs barking. Anyone who has visited India will know that traffic noise is a way of life that starts early in the morning and continues as a living, breathing annoyance well into the night.

It's amazing how, with time and practice, it becomes easier to control the Monkey Mind and get into a deep meditative state, even with such random noise as traffic. After years of practice I find I am happier meditating with sounds around me and using instruments than meditating in total silence. I can meditate in 4WDs, trains, buses and even planes, using the sound and the vibration to help take me away.

The thing I have found while teaching meditation is that people still come back to me and ask how to deal with the Monkey Mind because, when they take a few breaths, the mind goes off again – like people's frustration in peak hour traffic.

The easiest way I know to deal with this is to start meditating with a pad and pen handy. Sit at a table and start the mediation process as outlined in exercise one.

Allow yourself to relax. When a thought comes into your mind – such as the fact you need to do the shopping – acknowledge that thought and say thank you to the universe. If the thought pops back into your mind, write it down on the pad. Take yourself back into a meditative state and as other things pop into your mind recognise them and if they pop back in again write them down.

When I first started to meditate I would find that a whole list of things would float through my consciousness. Not only shopping, I found I was planning my day, my week, and so on. It was frustrating until I worked out it was more productive to accept these conscious thoughts and then move on.

A tip is to recognise that in the beginning, your whole ten minutes may be taken up with Monkey Mind thoughts. It is important to understand that this is a normal part of learning to meditate. So don't give up. Try it again the following day as each time Monkey Mind will lessen. By acknowledging the conscious Monkey Mind you control it. You give yourself permission to relax and free yourself of the distracting thoughts for future meditations.

With time, patience and practice, instead of coming up with a list of things to do when you are not meditating, you will find yourself able to meditate on a progressively deeper level and achieve a better state of overall wellbeing.

Another phenomenon that occurs while learning to meditate is body consciousness. In simple terms we train our minds and bodies to be busy and active all day every day, so when we want it to sit still the body starts to complain. This might start with an itch around the face before moving onto a pain between the shoulders. Legs might feel tingly and so on. The only way I know to deal with this is to breathe your way through it.

In essence, breathing through the body consciousness is your way of telling your body that it's okay to relax. Like quieting the Monkey Mind, this does take time, patience, persistence and practice to overcome.

Sound via any means, and – more especially – an instrument of some description, will let you break through Monkey Mind and Body Consciousness by providing a focus for mind and body to work together to achieve the ultimate aim of creating a happier, healthier mind and body.

Exercise 1

Following the Breath

There are many ways to bring about a meditative, peaceful state within the body. The best way I know, which can be done anywhere and anytime, is by using the breath to create a sound that allows you to reach a blissful awareness of self and the universe. This exercise is also a great way to replenish energy lost during our busy lives.

Find a seat – inside or out – and get comfortable, sitting as upright as possible. Place both feet flat on the ground. Very gently allow your eyelids to close and take a few deep breaths in through the nose and out through the mouth.

The reason for closing your eyes gently is that if you jam them shut and hold them tightly closed, you are forcing your mind to think about them. If your eyes are open then it will be easier to get distracted by movement in your vision. Gently closed is more natural and creates a more relaxed state to meditate in.

Very gently move your head forwards and backwards while taking some deep breaths. Slowly move your head from side to side while continuing to take deep breaths. Breathing should continue to be in through the nose and out through the mouth. After doing this a few times breathe deeply into your stomach, then roll your shoulders backwards and forwards gently as you breathe out.

After doing this, continue to breathe in and out while saying under your breath, 'It's okay to relax. It's okay to have this time for me.' This is important as you have to consciously and subconsciously give yourself permission to relax. At this point, place your hands on your legs, palms down.

With no sounds other than those in your environment, take a deep breath in through the nose and while listening to the sound of the breath moving in through the nose and down into the pit of your stomach, visualise the air trail flowing through this cycle.

Get a sense of the air swirling around inside the bottom of your diaphragm, then allow the breath to be expelled from your lungs through your mouth at a controlled rate. Pursing your lips slightly will create a sound and also help control the exhalation of the air on the outward breath. This will allow you to follow the sound of the air with your ears and your consciousness.

Follow the air until it stops and becomes silent. Wait for three seconds, then repeat the process.

As you get better at this, you will find yourself breathing in deeply and holding for the count of three before expelling the air through the mouth.

The idea is to repeat this process for five minutes initially each day for a week or two, then build up to ten, then fifteen minutes or longer over weeks and months – as long as you need to in order to achieve a sense of peace within the mind and energy within the body.

With practice, this simple exercise will allow oxygen to flow more freely through the body, which produces several health benefits such as helping to remove carbon dioxide – a natural waste product of the body.

Deep breathing also helps oxygenate the blood, muscles and brain, relieving tension and stress, which is another positive to practice meditation. These are just a few benefits.

While the breath work is one part of the process, the sound and vibration caused by the movement of air creates the focus for the mind, thus helping to create a relaxed state of being.

The hard part, as with all meditation regardless of the style, is that the Monkey Mind tries to stop you. As mentioned earlier it takes some time and practice to control the Monkey Mind.

Time, however, equals love and love promotes healing. It's worth allowing yourself at least five minutes a day to love and heal yourself.

Exercise 2

Following the Sound

The next exercise requires getting yourself into a relaxed state as per exercise one, then using an instrument such as a crystal bowl, drum, rattle or even a CD with specific sounds.

Meditating with an instrument is very effective as it creates a stronger vibration through the body than just simple breathing, and gives your mind a focus to work with, which also helps manage the Monkey Mind.

Once you get into that beautiful relaxed space as per exercise one, strike your instrument once gently. Allow yourself to hear the sound and feel the vibration. With your conscious mind following the sound, allow your body to feel the vibration resonate within you.

Strike it again and open your mind to the healing properties of the sound reverberating through your body from one end to the other. With your eyes closed it's very normal to see colour associated with the sound.

Allow this to work with you as well. With time and practice this will allow you to become very focused on all aspects of the meditation and you will drift off into a blissful state.

I suggest playing the instrument at your own leisure at this point. Play fast, play strong, play softly and dreamily. Your body and mind will create what feels right for you at that particular point in time, which I refer to as the *here and now*!

If you are playing an instrument that allows you to move around – such as a drum – and you feel the need to stand up and dance while drumming, then do it.

Sway gently or move fast and allow your subconscious connection to your body to take over and let yourself become active and energetic to achieve the best mental and physical state possible.

The aim behind this exercise is to trust your intuition by listening to your body and what it needs regarding sound and vibration. By following this process you will get the most out of your healing experience. In rounding out this chapter, vibrational healing starts on a cellular level from the start of our lives as an energetic being with a physical body, until we cross over in to the spirit world and revert back to being an energetic being without a physical body. In our physical lives energy, sound and colour vibrations define us in all ways, from the clothes we wear to the music we love.

In fact, sound and colour are a vital part of our physical existence on this planet. Why not go out and enhance your life with sound, vibration and colour and see how many people you can inspire with your exuberance for a healthy mind and a healthy life!

Some Interesting Facts

An ABC Science report by Kathy Graham, published 18 May 2006, reports that hearing is the last sense to fail before death. Dr Katherine Clark, a staff specialist in palliative care at Royal Prince Alfred Hospital, Sydney, is familiar with the common symptoms experienced by people on their deathbed.

She clarifies:

> 'Of course, each person's death is unique, so you might see only some of these symptoms or none of them.'

According to Clark, a person in the last stages of life will typically sleep more. Even so, loved ones are encouraged to keep talking to them.

> 'There's research based on electroencephalograms (EEGs) of people's brainwaves that indicates hearing is the last sense to go.'

It's a fascinating story to read.

There is some amazing evidence extolling the virtues of vibrational healing and sound. There is so much information available on the internet that it's mind blowing.

Having trolled through various vibrational healing sites on the web, such as the San Francisco-based Globe Institute – Sound & Consciousness site, I extracted a few facts verbatim to consider.

People in a coma have often reported they could hear, even though their brain was in a very deep state of consciousness with very little activity occurring within the brain.

Our brainwaves can be measured in Hertz. The measurements below indicate that, in a deep meditative state, our consciousness allows us to 'hear' and experience soundwaves at a much lower level than in an awake state.

By slowing things down we shut down the mind chatter and, therefore, heal on a deeper level.

- Gamma Waves – Heightened Perception – 14 to 40 Hz
- Beta Waves – Wakefulness – 14 to 40 Hz
- Alpha Waves – Relaxation & Meditation – 8 to 13Hz
- Delta Waves – Deep Sleep – 0.5 to 3Hz
- Theta Waves – Deep Dreaming & Meditation – 4 to 7Hz

Here are some quotes with some very interesting titbits from the Globe Institute – Sound & Consciousness website:

- Doctors have found that if a patient listens to thirty minutes a day of their favourite music, it does more than relax them mentally – it also benefits them physically by expanding and clearing blood vessels. It is believed to work by triggering the release into the bloodstream of nitric oxide, which helps to prevent the build-up of blood clots and harmful cholesterol.
- A Brazilian study found that Mozart's music improved patients' performance in a sight test aimed at checking peripheral vision of people with glaucoma.
- According to a paper in the *Journal of Advanced Nursing*, listening to music can reduce chronic pain by up to 21 per cent. It can also make people feel more in control of their pain and less disabled by their condition.
- According to a study in the *Journal of Advanced Nursing*, repeating mantras can help control the symptoms of post-traumatic stress disorder, have a calming effect in traffic and even ease the boredom of exercise.
- A project led by a researcher from the University of Western Sydney has found that music therapy can help

- sick babies in intensive care maintain normal behavioural development, making them less irritable, upset, and less likely to cry.
- The binaural-beat appears to be associated with an electroencephalographic (EEG) frequency-following response in the brain. Many studies have demonstrated the presence of a frequency-following response to auditory stimuli, recorded at the vertex of the human brain (top of the head). This EEG activity was termed 'frequency-following response' because its period corresponds to the fundamental frequency of the stimulus (Smith, Marsh, & Brown, 1975).
- Certain musical components in Mozart's music have been shown in research to activate the brain-enhancing learning processes.

publisher

The Written Word as Therapy

Blaise van Hecke

What is truer than truth? The story.

This Jewish proverb gets to the heart of what it means to be human. Through story we can learn the truth about ourselves and the world around us and make sense of what we can't understand.

It is debated that dis-ease is often created in the mind, so if there is a way to address it, we can go a long way to being dis-ease free. Reading and writing are both well-used therapies to treat such maladies as depression, anxiety, stress and the onset of dementia.

I have always been enchanted by stories. When I was about seven, radio serials enthralled me. I'd sit outside with our little transistor, fiddling with the dials to get a clear signal, holding my breath in anticipation.

A rich, deep English voice would seduce me and I was transported to the land of *Watership Down* (Richard Adams, 1972).

This is where I learnt about the power of story.

It didn't matter that I was hearing a story about rabbits – in fact, that was more exciting because it fed my imagination.

I learnt about social relationships, loyalty, survival, community and resilience, and that you should never underestimate the little guy (sorry, rabbit). That's a lot to put before a seven-year-old in one story, but I absorbed it effortlessly.

As soon as I was able to read, I would devour everything I could get my hands on. Books were my way out into the world at a time when TV was less prevalent and there was no such thing as social media. While my brothers were play wrestling with each other (also an important part of childhood), I was finding out about the lost land of Atlantis or gripped by the mystery in the *Famous Five*.

Books are awesome. They're good for you. But if statistics show us that only 46% of Australians have decent literacy skills, then many people are missing out on the magic of books.

This is why I feel compelled to spread the joy of reading to the masses and just about all the work I do is centred on it. Without good literacy skills, people have less job opportunities and this has a flow-on effect on self-esteem and life quality.

Recently I read in the *Herald Sun* that reading for as little as six minutes can reduce your current stress by 68%. As you can imagine, I pointed this out to my other half as justification for how much I read. But there are so many other good reasons to read a book.

Ever heard the term 'use it or lose it'? It applies to all parts of our body, including the brain. Reading is good mental stimulation and can slow or prevent the onset of Alzheimer's disease and dementia.

So while you're using reading as a health benefit, you can also increase your knowledge from both non-fiction and fiction books.

Don't think a novel has no knowledge to impart. Writers spend a lot of time researching their facts to put in their stories. We should never stop learning and reading allows us to keep doing it.

Best of all, reading is fun! A reader can be transported to a totally different world or be educated about a topic that interests them and even subjects that they know nothing about.

In my working life, surrounded by books, I have seen the evidence of how reading can affect a person's life and that there seems to be overwhelming evidence that literacy skills have a direct link to a person's happiness and success: economic status, aspirations, family life, health and community engagement.

Imagine not having the literacy skills to be able to perform the most basic functions, such as read a bus timetable, the instructions on a medicine bottle, or to write a resume.

Being able to perform these tasks fulfil basic needs. The more people in our community without these skills, the less resilient we are.

As a community, we need to make sure that each person is given the skills to increase their chances of an improvement in life. The better equipped we are for the basic things, the more we can grow and tackle the more extreme events that might come our way.

It is part of the human condition to experience suffering of some kind. These sufferings can be extremes: love, hate, loneliness, disease, joy and exaltation. How we deal with these extremes will determine how resilient we are, how happy or content we are, or even how miserable we are.

It is also part of being human that we share stories and connect with each other. Through stories we can exchange experiences, help each other and grow as humans. We have been doing this for thousands of years and will continue to do so far into the future.

Bibliotherapy (reading as therapy) is not a new idea and my feelings about it are not revolutionary. My own reading experiences have shaped my life.

Reading helps me get to sleep, relaxes me, captivates me and makes me a happier, more empathetic person. Can you read yourself happy? I believe you can.

The ancient Egyptians considered a library a 'house of healing for the soul'. Walking into a library or bookshop can have a calming affect on people. The use of books to change behaviour and reduce stress dates back to the Middle Ages.

In the 19th century, doctors and psychiatric nurses prescribed everything from the Bible to travel literature as therapy for an unsettled mind. A quick look at Google will take you to resources on the kinds of books that will help you deal with certain maladies such as depression, anxiety and dementia – remedies, if you like, for what ails your mind.

Reading both fiction and non-fiction sharpens analytical thinking, social ability, empathy and imagination as well as a sense of morality.

Most of these things are covered in that simple little story, *Watership Down*, a book that was written to entertain the author's children.

Here are ten ways that reading is good for your mind:

1. Provides mental stimulation
This will depend on the reading matter. Both fiction and non-fiction can be stimulating, but if you pick up a romance novel that could be stimulating in different ways!

2. Reduces stress
The act of reading brings the reader into the present moment. This immediately reduces stress as everything outside of the 'reading bubble' is pushed away for at least the time of reading. The content of the book can further add to this depending on the subject matter.

3. Increases knowledge
This is very obvious but any book will allow the reader to learn something, whether it is about relationships between characters in a novel or the history of WWII.

4. Increases vocabulary
The more we read, the more unfamiliar words we come across. Even if the reader doesn't look up these words in the dictionary, often the meaning can be gleaned from the context of the sentence.

5. Improves memory
This is simply by the fact that the more we use that muscle called the brain, the stronger, faster, more amazing it becomes.

6. Increases analytical skills
The more we do something, the better we get at it. Reading continually uses the brain, allowing it to not only ask more questions but to get more answers.

7. Improves concentration
It stands to reason that the more we read, the more we are using our grey matter. This is why reading is considered a valuable tool to help people fend off the onset of dementia or avoid it altogether. More study is being conducted in this area but it won't hurt to heed the suggestions that it might help.

8. Improves writing skills
The more we read, the more we understand the rhythm of sentences, the nuances of the author's voice and the rules of grammar. I always tell writers that you cannot expect to improve your writing craft if you are not a reader yourself.

9. It's calming
There is nothing like going to bed with a good book to get you in the mood for sleep. Or reading a book to a child to get them to sit still for a while.

10. Is entertaining

We read, write, watch movies and listen to music for the pure enjoyment of story. Every reader has their own kind of story that they like and none is better than the other if it creates the same level of entertainment and wellbeing in a person. One reader might love to read only romance novels while another might like the thrill of a *whodunit*.

Reading is mostly a solitary pastime and it can feel isolating. A great way to take your reading to the next level is to join a book group. I have been a part of a book group for ten years. During this time, we have read some great books and some average books. The best part of being in this group is that we are a mix of people with different experiences and opinions. When we read and discuss a book, it opens up a dialogue that might never happen in other situations.

I have talked to many people who are part of a book group and they say things like, 'It's so great to be able to discuss how I felt when a character did this or that and to see how others reacted to it', or 'I was abused as a teenager. We had a book that dealt with this topic and I was able to be part of the discussion without revealing my past. It helped me a lot to hear how others perceived the situation and that I was not to blame for what happened. I had carried this secret for years and I was able to open up about it'.

These are powerful but gentle ways for people to heal along with the sense of community and sharing that goes with being part of any social group.

The other side to story is the writing of them. Reading and writing go hand in hand, both being creative expressions. Humans are spiritual beings and writing can be a potent form of meditation that connects us mind, body and soul.

I attended an author event one wintery evening at my local library. As a reader and a writer I am always interested in the person behind the story and what makes them tick. This particular evening, Australian author Barry Heard was guest speaker. Barry was conscripted in Australia's first national service ballot and served in Vietnam. Twenty years after returning from Vietnam, Barry suffered a breakdown due to post-traumatic stress disorder.

Part of the recovery for Barry was to attend group therapy sessions with other Vietnam Vets. These sessions were excruciating for the men who had spent years suffering in silence. Slowly they began to express themselves and heal. What Barry found most useful was when his therapist suggested that he write about his experiences by writing a letter to himself about what he was feeling. Once he started, he couldn't stop. What he wrote became his award-winning book, *Well Done, Those Men*.

At question time, I asked Barry if he thought that writing it down saved him. He nodded enthusiastically. 'Yes, it was like I had verbal diarrhoea, it felt like I was writing myself well!' This gave me goose bumps because I feel this about words – they can be life-saving. Not only did the writing help him to heal, but many other Vietnam vets told him that reading his book helped them a great deal also.

The use of writing as therapy is not to produce an outstanding literary work of art (or bestselling book), but to concentrate on the emotional expression, to articulate unexpressed and unexplored feelings. Barry and so many other war vets had done the silent thing for twenty years. It's no wonder that they had an emotional meltdown at some stage. There is only so long that you can keep a lid on something before it will explode. Writing gives meaningful expression to something that hasn't been, or cannot be spoken aloud. It's a way for the writer to say what is pent up in their head and heart in a very safe way. This can be a bridge to articulating something aloud.

Just think about a time when you might have been angry about something. If you had the chance to verbalise your anger, and felt safe, would you just spew the words out? Most likely you would. Many people do. But if you don't feel safe, writing them down is a good way to get them out without saying something to someone that you might regret.

Ask most writers about why they write and many will tell you that it's because they need to make sense of what is in their head. It's a compulsion and many do not feel 'right' until they get what is in their head out onto the page. But writing isn't just for writers. It is a strong, therapeutic practice, a way to observe thoughts and feelings and help track spinning thoughts. Writing is speaking to another consciousness or another part of our self. This is how we create a mind-body-spirit connection. The page is an anonymous therapist, a safe place to expose and explore ourselves.

For me, the need to write builds up. If I don't write when it builds up, the safety valve won't hold. If I leave it too long I get agitated and mean about things around me. I guess it must be like running for some people, or even sex. It's a release.

Journal writing is one of the most effective and easy ways to use writing as therapy. My bookshelves are littered with pretty journals that I have used in a haphazard way. There is most likely no chronological order to these notebooks, although there is one that I used consistently over about fifteen years. I will admit that I use my journal more when I am unhappy or struggling with things. When I'm happy, I don't have the *need* to write.

Consequently, if someone were to read them, they might get the impression that I have been more miserable throughout my life than I have been. These journals have a lot of mundane jottings too, like details about the weather, what my kids were doing or how tired I was. Scattered amongst these mundane entries, though, are plenty of descriptions of the blessings in my life like slipping into freshly laundered sheets, the health of my two boys or the antics of our dog as a puppy.

Journal writing is a place where you can download. To do this you need to write freely and without censorship. This is not the time to worry about what you are writing, how grammatically correct it is or who else might read it. I thought about including some entries from my journals here but because they are uncensored, and contain names of family and friends, I decided against it. None of those entries were intended to be read by anyone other than myself and to share them actually feels like I am sharing my own secrets, cheating on myself, strange as that sounds.

Write whatever is on your mind. Sometimes there might not be much to say. Maybe you can just record some of the everyday events that happen, or express gratitude for what you did or have. You'd be surprised how much better it makes you feel to note down what you are grateful for. It will put your life in perspective, especially for people in a country like Australia where we are so fortunate. Even writing about your own strengths, or your proud moments, will help you to lift your mood and empower yourself.

The simple act of journaling is very powerful. I'm not actually sure why, but the physical act of writing it down (and I strongly suggest that the journal be handwritten) seems to help the writer process a problem. It's a safe way to get it out of your head by 'telling' your problems to your *therapist* (yourself or the paper). This can then create a bridge between yourself and the unsayable. By voicing it, you are making it real, not just thoughts swirling around in your head. By writing these thoughts down you may find that they become more ordered. You may even find that you unearth answers when you ask questions.

Here's an example of how writing it down will help you: if you tend to be a person who rarely says 'no' when asked for a favour, over time you start to feel used and abused and maybe even become angry at yourself for allowing others to use and abuse you. Maybe you're not even aware of the fact that you are 'allowing' others to use you. You might just think that people see you as a pushover. But if you write about these events, you will start to see that there is a pattern, or that you are repeating a behaviour. In the writing about it, you may also find that you come up with a solution for yourself to change your own behaviour. By simply writing, 'I don't want to be a "yes" person anymore because I am exhausted. I will find a way to change this', you will find that the answer comes to you (maybe not straight away) because you've manifested it.

It is useful to write daily in a journal, ideally at the end of the day. Make it part of your routine. This way, it can become a way of downloading or debriefing and will help you sleep better by parking all of your day onto the page. If you can't think of something to write, simply write down three things that you are grateful for. Or, you could write down your problem as a question and jot down some possible solutions. You might find by morning that you have solved your dilemma.

If you're feeling more creative, writing poetry can also be very therapeutic. You don't have to be a dedicated poet. Just enjoy playing with words and imagery. For instance, you could try making a list of positive images from your childhood (or a good time in your life). Then write down some emotions that you associate with those images. Using the five senses (six if you're so inclined), create a poem from the images and emotions that you've gathered. You might be surprised with what you come up with.

If you have a particular problem with a person, a well-used endeavour is to write a letter. You could do this within your journal writing, but you might find it more powerful to write a real letter with the intention of not delivering it. The idea of writing a letter is to have a conversation with this person that you wish you could have in real life. It might be about how they make you feel, how you wish they would forgive you for something (explaining yourself) or how you forgive them for something. Just like a verbal tirade might let off steam and make you feel better, writing how you feel in a letter will do the same. The difference is that the latter is more measured and less volatile.

The mind is a wonderfully complex structure, much of its capacity still unknown. Of course it works in conjunction with other organs and structures within our body and is therefore not working in isolation, so we cannot give it all the credit for the state of our health and wellbeing. We need to feed it with things that will keep it healthy and in good working order: good nutrition and exercise. In addition, we need to feed it with ideas and thoughts that elevate us to a higher state of being. We can't do that if we are in a state of confusion, distress or even ignorance. The written word can go a long way to improving our development and emotional wellbeing, which in turn can diminish any state of dis-ease.

counsellor

Creating and Maintaining a Healthy Mind

Dr Talia Steed

As a doctor and counsellor, and as someone who's been through their own share of mental challenges, I feel that the cultivation of a healthy mind is the foundation for living a rich, meaningful and wholehearted life.

I started out as a medical doctor in a world completely unsuited to my personality. This experience – in combination with other outside world challenges and inside battles of the mind – lead me to a very difficult place, which I have been fortunate to leave behind. From these personal experiences, my medical years as a trainee in Psychiatry, and thereafter as a counsellor, I have witnessed that it is the ability to look within and shift entrenched thought and emotional patterns that creates the possibility of a whole new way of operating in our outside worlds.

I also believe in a holistic approach to wellbeing that encompasses Body, Mind and Spirit, as each are intricately linked. When we can unite all the parts of us that tend to become disconnected and fragmented through life, it is a step towards becoming integrated and whole. From this place of wholeness, we can develop contentment, peace and joy within our lives. Our outside world is a reflection of our world within, so each and every one of us has the power to make our life a beautiful, joyous adventure.

The following sections are excerpts from my

book that I hope share some of what has helped me cultivate and maintain a mind that is not just healthy, but a life filled with vitality, wellbeing and joy.

My wish for you, the reader, is to find ways that you too can shift your life around and develop acceptance and love for all aspects that constitute who you are as a person.

Body
Body love
Our body is the vessel that houses our inner soul. I believe there are two very important aspects as to how we conceptualise it.

Firstly, nurture.

We show ourselves respect by taking care of our body, which involves using the right fuel to sustain it and keeping it active to maintain its function. It is important to consume produce that is not simply 'healthy' by some person's definition of the day, but nutritious and energy-enhancing. Eating in this way contributes to the vitality of not only our physical self, but also our mind and spirit.

The impact of what we put into our body on our mood, as well as our levels of anxiety and irritability, is significant. Our mental health suffers when we miss out on certain key elements essential to our wellbeing. We foster mental wellbeing and vitality through our diet by keeping it varied. When we make restrictions on what we allow into our body, we are making it more sensitive to the effects of different foods when we are later exposed to them. This is why so many people have developed intolerances to different food groups. We need to expose the body to a variety of foods to keep up its ability to process a wide proportion of them.

The other important concept related to how we think about our bodies is impermanence. I once had a very imprinting experience during my medical days when I witnessed the preparations for an orthopaedic surgery on a very old lady. Just before the commencement of the procedure, she lay there on the operating table fully anaesthetised. The surgeons proceeded to move her limbs into the most suitable position to operate. I had a very strong reaction to this scenario as it made me contemplate my own mortality.

Of course, rationally, I am aware, as most of us are, about the process of life and ageing, but I had been living in a state of denial, as many people often do. At that moment I had a strong gut realisation that everyone gets old – if they survive and are lucky enough to make it there. Reminding myself of this experience over the years has helped me remember the futility of trying to reach the version each of us creates of our 'perfect' body and the impermanence of our life in both the physical and mental form.

Mind
Authenticity and awareness of self
Authenticity is to live genuinely, honestly, and in alignment with our true characteristics and self. It may seem like an easy principle. In reality, it is much more difficult to put into practice. This

is often because we can go for many years not knowing who we really are and what we stand for. When we aren't sure of ourselves and our place in the world, it is difficult to live in an authentic way.

Inauthentic living can manifest in our lives in our actions and the choices we make. We may engage in the wrong relationship, go down a career path unsuited to our self, or implement repetitive unhelpful behaviours in our daily life. Many people also use maladaptive coping strategies to deal with the impact of inauthentic living, such as alcohol, drugs, food or sex. This may help us in the short-term to avoid addressing underlying issues, but in the long-term can lead us into a downward spiral that becomes increasingly difficult to make our way out of.

The way in which we can access authenticity and begin to make changes in our lives is through awareness, which is the development of a deeper understanding of our self. Through this process, we come to learn who we actually are as a person, and *not* who our parents, society, or even *we* had wanted ourselves to be. Initially, feelings of disappointment may arise in the discovery that we are not the right fit for something we thought we wanted in our life. This can feel despairing, discouraging, and demoralising that we do not have the necessary qualities.

With time and the development of greater self-awareness and insight, we can develop an understanding of all characteristics – both positive and negative – that constitute who we are as a whole. Using this knowledge, we can focus on expanding and developing our natural skill set, and set out to find our place in this world.

When we free our minds and hearts, and proceed with an open, and genuine attitude, opportunities arise to lead us in new directions. With greater self-awareness we discover possibilities in life that we had never considered before.

Once we are living an authentic life aligned with our true values and purpose, the most surprising discovery often occurs when we look back and can't imagine our life having turned out any differently.

The Impact of Isolation on the Mind

Isolation is one of the biggest predictors for becoming depressed. Humans are social beings who thrive when relating with others. This is true whether we are extroverts who need prolonged time in the company of others, or introverts who need less, but still benefit from frequent, shorter interactions.

When we spend extended periods of time on our own, our mood can become flat and down. Signs that the isolation may be affecting us more deeply include losing our sense of motivation to do things and a reduced sense of enjoyment in things that we generally have enjoyed.

We may also begin to experience a disrupted sleep pattern with either the desire to sleep more and throughout the day. Waking very early and being unable to get back to sleep is often a sign that something is not quite as it should be.

Sometimes our appetite changes, where we either lose the desire to eat or compensate for our loneliness and despair by eating more.

We can experience feelings of severe fatigue, finding it difficult to do even the basic tasks of showering, preparing a meal, or reading a book.

Sometimes we can also become highly anxious, feeling on edge, unable to wind down, and become restless, and agitated.

We may become aware of our heart racing, feeling short of breath, having more frequent headaches and stomach aches, and a multitude of other physical symptoms.

Sometimes when these changes go on for an extended time, we begin to feel helpless to make changes and hopeless about our future being any brighter.

This can lead to thoughts of not wanting to be alive and is a sign that our body, mind and spirit are in need of something we are not getting from our current life situation.

This is why it is so important to take care of ourselves both physically and mentally.

We all have different things that work for us, but some of the things that I believe we can do to keep our spirits up and prevent a decline into prolonged negative emotional states include the following:

Physically

- **Regular exercise**: this helps to keep us energised and uplifted, whether we are regular walkers, runners, swimmers or yogis. Whatever it is that you are drawn to is what you should keep up with.

- **Being aware of your alcohol consumption**: it is so easy to fall into the trap of drinking more when going through a difficult time or in attempt to shift a negative mood state. However, alcohol has a depressant effect and can exacerbate low mood and/or anxiety. It can also precipitate these feelings in those of us not currently feeling down or anxious.

Mentally

- **Socialising**: it is so important to maintain a social network. The amount and frequency of this varies for us all, but we all need to have some contact with others as social human beings. If you are someone with few family members or friends, getting involved in community events can be helpful. Even volunteering your time to do something for others can be an uplifting experience.
- **Meditation**: this is something that is always useful in cultivating wellbeing and inner peace. We can do this anywhere, alone, or in the company of others. When we unite with like-minded people it can have a deeper and more profound impact on our psyche. Yoga, Tai Chi and Pilates are just some of the other more active practices that incorporate this element of mindful meditative practice.

When we are focused and engaged in any activity it can be a form of meditation, even for those of us who normally shy away from formal mediation practices.

And, in difficult times, always remember that *This Too Shall Pass*.

Nothing is fixed and life is about constant flux and change. If you are deeply suffering, please let someone know and reach out for help.

Spirit
Spirituality

This is something that I find challenging to write about, as it is a unique and individual experience for each of us. Our spiritual path is about embarking on a journey within. When we listen to our instincts and truly connect to our true, essential self, we can reach that place of awareness, understanding, faith and trust in the universe, and our place within it.

Since childhood I have always been a person who was spiritually inclined. From an early age, I questioned the meaning of our human existence and the religious way of thinking I was exposed to. Over the years, though, with more 'pressing' external experiences demanding my attention, my internal questioning subsided. I lost touch with this aspect of myself, which was rediscovered out of necessity and survival following my decline into depression.

Since that time, I have recommenced the pursuit of my inner spiritual growth and have found that this is something that helps me put my life and struggles into perspective. I know that I am just a tiny being amongst an infinite universe – as we all are – and that one day, in a relatively short period of time, my life in this human body will cease to exist. I believe that my purpose here in this life is for my soul to grow and evolve, and learn the lessons meant for my unique being in this lifetime.

I think that exploring a spiritual path is something that each one of us can embark upon, to develop a stronger inner core. By cultivating our inner power and resilience, we each have the capacity to withstand the adversities and challenges we encounter in our external worlds.

Mindfulness and Meditation

So often people associate meditation with emptying one's mind of thoughts but this is probably an impossible task for most of us. Mindfulness meditation teaches us that the aim is not to remove thoughts from our mind, because thought is what the human mind has evolved to do. Instead, the aim is to develop an awareness of thought, to watch our mind and strengthen the observer self within us beneath the ever-changing and chaotic-thinking mind.

In a Mindful Breathing practice, for example, we start by focusing our attention on our breath. When thoughts come up, as they inevitably will, we observe these thoughts, noticing that our attention has drifted, and then in a calm, non-judgmental way, refocus our attention on the breath. This seemingly simple but often very challenging practice has the capability to reduce the level of distress from heightened and uncomfortable emotional states. It may not eliminate the negative feelings or experiences, but it can help us endure them.

The benefits of this practice are much more noticeable when we practise these skills in a calm frame of mind, as when we are in the most heightened state of arousal it's much more difficult for anything to be of benefit. A regular meditation practice helps us reduce the likelihood of becoming so distressed in the first place and gives us the best chance of coping with such negative emotional states when they arise.

Integration and Discovering Your True Purpose

Often we go through periods in our life in which we feel lost, stuck or unable to choose a path to follow. Sometimes this can manifest in feeling flat, unmotivated or on edge for an extended period of time. If we can identify that we feel like this for a reason, though, we can use these uncomfortable feelings to actively make changes in our life that lead us in the direction we wish our life to take.

It is very hard in today's society to break free from the pressures and expectations of an achievement-focused world. There seems to be a general expectation that to be happy and fulfilled, there are criteria we need to meet. Firstly, we need to find meaningful and well-regarded work that reimburses us financially. However, not only should we work hard and generate a good income, we are also expected to have a content and happy family life, with strong, cohesive relationships; be social, and have a wide network of friends; live in a comfortable house; give back to the community;

maintain a healthy lifestyle; and have travelled widely. Instead of being appreciative and grateful for what we do have, this pressure leads to many becoming dissatisfied when even one of these domains is lacking.

In one of my favourite books, *Tuesdays with Morrie* by Mitch Albom, Morrie says, 'The culture we have does not make people feel good about themselves. And you have to be strong enough to say if the culture doesn't work. Don't buy it.'

In order to find our true pathway and what will bring joy and happiness to our own life, we need to reject these messages and pursue whatever it is that makes us feel alive.

My good friend, Ian McTavish, in his book *A Prisoner's Wisdom*, quoted Gile Bailey who said, 'Don't ask yourself what the world needs. Ask yourself what makes you come alive and go and do that. Because what the world needs is more people who have come alive.'

Find what makes you feel excited, passionate and motivated. For some, this may not be what they do for work and they may view their occupation as simply their job. This is okay! They may have another passion in life that their job allows them to pursue and enjoy.

Others may love spending time with close family or friends, but prefer not socialising with a wide circle of people, whilst there are some who prefer an active social life and work to minimize their alone time. What matters is that we are authentic in the way in which we live our life, because it is this that will bring contentment and satisfaction to us.

We need to live with acceptance and remove

the judgment we have of ourselves as best as we can. This can be a hard task when many of us have become such harsh critics of ourselves. The first step is awareness, as when we can stop, notice that harsh, inner voice, we can smile at our self and redirect our thinking.

I'd like to finish with a quote by one of my favourite authors, Brene Brown, who shows us how, through being vulnerable, living with awareness, and acting authentically, we can find true joy, love, and light in our lives ...

> 'Owning our story can be hard but not nearly as difficult as spending our lives running from it. Embracing our vulnerabilities is risky but not nearly as dangerous as giving up on love and belonging and joy – the experiences that make us the most vulnerable. Only when we are brave enough to explore the darkness will we discover the infinite power of our light.'

The Benefits of Kinesiology
Debbie Rossi

Kinesiology is the study of body movement and originated in the 1960s. The word 'kinesiology' comes from Greek:

kinesis = movement
logia = study.

Kinesiology is a complementary and energetic therapy that uses non-invasive muscle testing and body feedback to test your body for imbalances. These imbalances may be a result of nutritional deficiencies, hormonal imbalances, emotional upheaval, food sensitivities, structural misalignments, poor energy flow or negative self-beliefs. Kinesiology is one of the few complementary modalities that recognise the importance of body, mind and spirit in health and in healing.

My journey began with my daughter, who'd suffered recurring headaches from an early age. She was stuck in a cycle – pain-free, then headaches that would gradually worsen and lead to vomiting for about a day, then back to being pain-free for a few days. I tried in vain to help her and took her to many health professionals. We were never able to figure out why she was getting the headaches. I was treating her symptoms with painkillers, but never understanding their cause.

A friend who previously had a lot of success with

her kinesiologist suggested that her kinesiologist could help my daughter. Within one session, the kinesiologist had determined that dairy products were the reason for my daughter's headaches. I was not a big believer at this time, but there was nothing to lose, so I removed dairy products from her diet. Within three weeks the headaches had reduced dramatically, with no vomiting. Another three weeks later she was pain-free. She was like a different child – not only pain-free but she was no longer moody and seemed to be much happier within herself.

This experience evoked a desire to know how this had worked. I originally thought it was magic or that maybe the kinesiologist was psychic. I needed to learn how I could help my children by using these techniques. Hence, I enrolled in my Kinesiology course, at Kinesiology Schools Australia. And now, seven years later, I'm still amazed at what kinesiology can actually achieve for myself, my family and my clients.

Kinesiology is grounded in the study of anatomy and physiology, which was originally developed in the 1960s when Dr George Goodheart DC discovered that by using muscle testing you can gather information about the body. It was called 'Applied Kinesiology' and is still taught to chiropractors today, focusing on the muscle testing, Chinese medicine techniques, and energy flows around the body.

The energy flows around our bodies relate to muscles, organs, tissues and every cell that makes our body a living and feeling being. When this energy flow is interrupted due to emotional trauma, injury, nutritional or any other stressor, our whole body is affected. Often the energy flow will be blocked to certain parts of the body, therefore blocking the body's natural healing process. Kinesiology helps to identify and unblock the energy flows to allow the energy to flow freely once again. Acupressure massage, light touch and other simple correction techniques are then used to restore the energy flow of the whole body.

This type of energy balancing is also very effective in bringing a person closer to achieving a goal of their choice, in sport, relationships, learning, or life in general. It is through monitoring muscles that we can determine and implement changes in a person's life to enable them to be in alignment with their chosen goal.

Kinesiology monitors the movement of muscles in your body for feedback about what the body is going through. I like to explain it simply by saying that through muscle testing, your muscles will respond to something that is stressful to your body. For example, junk food will cause a muscle to have a weak response (since it is stressful for the body), whereas water will cause the muscle to have a strong response (since it is beneficial for the body).

The next logical question is, 'What is muscle testing and how do you test a muscle?' The human nervous system is designed to self-regulate and adapt to change. When we cannot adapt efficiently, the muscles will reflect the stress from the change in the central nervous system. And this stress creates specific muscle patterns that kinesiologists can assess using muscle-monitoring techniques.

The easiest way to understand this process is to think of the signals between the brain and the body as a feedback loop. As the brain adapts to the changes in the muscular system, the muscles signal the brain that the changes have taken place. It is a continual loop and your muscle will react either in a strong way or a weak way to what the brain is telling it.

Kinesiology deals with a lot of emotional issues in conjunction with a correction point around the body. Kinesiology uses pressure points and the meridian energy flow that is used in Traditional Chinese medicine. Also, different physical changes and changes in your environment will allow your muscles, and ultimately your body, to become strong and enhance the body's overall function.

My Kinesiology journey has helped me deal with many underlying emotions that have been brewing and bubbling away under the surface – my external persona – for many years. I had refused to look at these emotions because I was focusing on unimportant outside issues and not what was important on the inside. Kinesiology muscle testing helped me to test for answers to see these underlying emotions and belief patterns that I had set up in my life.

For many years, I suffered from headaches and lower back pain. These are the physical ailments that had been caused by my low self-worth, lack of self-belief, and a feeling that I'm not good enough, which came about as a result of bullying I experienced throughout my high school years. Through Kinesiology muscle testing, I have been able to pinpoint exactly what is going on, which has allowed me to work through my issues easier and quicker. Once you know the starting point, it is much easier to figure out what needs to change to make a long-lasting effect. Even now I use Kinesiology every day with myself and even my children. I find it to be a very valuable tool to use on a daily basis to keep myself in alignment with the present moment of being a happy and confident person.

Regular Kinesiology muscle testing helps maintain our body's equilibrium, healthy mind and emotional state. This enables us to be more at ease and handle the everyday emotional and environmental ups and downs. It is very important to have your body in a balanced and calm state on a daily basis. That way, when the ebbs and flows of life come, you are able to deal with them from a calm and balanced place.

There are a number of different exercise techniques that have been introduced into Kinesiology to help the mind and body to be at a balanced level, and to be calmer and more centred within. This is the aim of Kinesiology, because when you are in that balanced and centred state, your body will be able to deal with changes and heal itself from the inside out.

These exercises are called 'Brain Gym', which are physical exercises that a person does to stimulate brain activity. They are effective for both adults and children and are often used in the classroom environment to stimulate learning. In a Kinesiology session these brain exercises are essential in overcoming a negative past issue as our brain replays the old patterns over and over again. We need to reprogram our brain to work and think differently.

In recent brain studies it has been proven that, through repetition and patterns, our brain is pliable and changeable, which will support the brain to create new neural pathways. It is through incorporating these brain exercises that we can structurally realign our brain to more positive thinking, which therefore allows the changes to be easier and longer lasting.

In a Kinesiology session, you lie on your back on a massage table, fully clothed. An intention or goal is set for the session. This intention is what you want to work towards during the session. For example, 'I am committed to my health and fitness', or 'I respect and nurture myself every day.' This intention is set from discussions with you before the session begins.

Muscle testing is then used to discover which emotional patterns and emotional beliefs are at play. Whilst you discuss the emotions involved, the necessary corrections around your body will be made by using pressure points or a correction to the energy flow around your body.

Throughout the session, you will talk about your different emotional issues and a homework sheet will be prepared for you. This homework sheet will include the things that you have discussed during your session. It is for you to take away and complete so as to bring about changes in your everyday life.

Long-lasting changes are not going to happen in a single one-hour Kinesiology session. These changes take time and practice to incorporate into every day and routines. Often, our negative thought patterns, behaviours and emotions take on a life of their own and run on automatic to the point where we do not even know how much they are affecting our lives.

When this happens they have become so ingrained that they become our way of life. The homework you are given will empower you with the tools to break these old habits. It takes twenty-eight days to break an old habit and re-program our thoughts and feelings into a more positive and life affirming-way of thinking.

Homework may be something as simple as saying an affirmation every day or introducing a new thought pattern. It may be a brain exercise that needs to be incorporated into your life. It may be a change in outlook or perspective of life. It could also be a physical change in your environment or diet.

I practise Kinesiology every day in my life. I often use self-muscle testing. For example, if I have a back ache, I will use muscle testing to test why I have the back ache and why I let this back ache come into my life.

Rather than dealing with the back ache itself, I ask, 'What do I need to deal with to get rid of my back ache?' I always look at the underlying issue. What is the emotional cause or reason? When I can understand the cause for my back ache and deal with it, nine times out of ten my back ache will go.

This is what I teach my clients through Kinesiology. They always need to look at the underlying reason why something has happened in their life. There is no point looking at the symptoms; you need to look at the cause. Sometimes, when you are not looking at the cause of the symptom, you use a Band-Aid fix and start a cycle, like my daughter when she was young.

We always need to go back to what was the origin of the problem and not look at those outside things that are happening. Look at the issue itself and make sure you fix it from that beginning point, not from the end result.

Kinesiology is a powerful tool. It cuts through and gets right into the core issues. Dealing with these issues is ultimately the only way to grow and develop in life. In my experience with myself and my clients I have noticed that we continue to think, react and act the same way based on the same thought patterns, which are a result of past negative experiences.

It becomes a continual loop of the same thoughts and feelings, which we do not even realise are occurring. Which means that we will not be able to break the cycle until we acknowledge what the originating causes and thought patterns are. At the end of the day, you cannot change what you do not acknowledge.

It is about focusing on your inner thoughts and feelings. Do I have low self-worth or low self-love? Do I have low confidence? How can I build myself up from the inside? This is how to make long-lasting changes to your life, by focusing on the things inside that you can change.

When we concentrate on the outside issue we lose our focus and do not deal with the internal issues. The outside issue is only a reflection of your internal thoughts or feelings. This is why Kinesiology is beneficial as a way to find and address inner issues so that we move past them and into all that our lives have to offer.

Many clients I see lack a basic fundamental self-love and self-worth. Many times I hear from my clients that *if only I had a new job* or *if only I was invited out with friends* or *if only I lost weight* 'then I would be happy'. These *if onlys* are sometimes not within our immediate control and leave a person feeling angry, frustrated and depressed.

It does not matter which job you have, if you're socially accepted, or how much you weigh as you will be the same person with the same thoughts, insecurities and worries regardless of the situation. By looking away from these *if onlys* we can focus on what is important, improving our self-love and becoming the person we can feel proud of and be happy with.

I know this to be true with not only my clients but also myself as I was once this person looking for answers and quick-fixes. This is often the easy path to take, as it is easier to change jobs or lose weight rather than deal with the real internal emotions of life. Here, in these real emotions, is where we can find peace and self-acceptance within ourselves to reflect into our everyday lives.

One of the problems with Kinesiology is that people get confused or overwhelmed with the muscle-testing techniques. Here is a simple system that is easy to learn and apply without anyone noticing what you are doing.

The advantages are:
1. You can test yourself in a reliable way.
2. It is discreet. People will not stare at you or wonder what you are doing.
3. You can test yourself in this way at a shopping centre with bags in your hands.
4. You can do this at home to maintain your Kinesiology balances.
5. You can teach your children this.

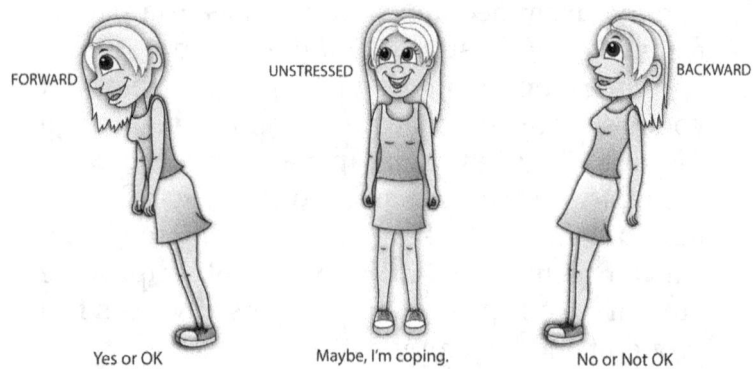

FORWARD — Yes or OK
UNSTRESSED — Maybe, I'm coping.
BACKWARD — No or Not OK

Basic versions

Leaning Forward	Body Upright	Leaning Back
Drawn to	Unstressed	Repelled by
I'm doing well	Just coping	Not coping
Yes	Maybe	No
Okay	Hanging in	Not okay
Moving forward	No progress	Moving away
Positive	Static	Negative

What Can I Test?

The possibilities are endless of what you can test using the whole body testing method. I would recommend that you only test simple and easy things to begin with and continue with your regular Kinesiology sessions with a qualified kinesiologist to keep your whole body testing on track.

I would like to emphasise the point here that Kinesiology does not diagnose medical conditions. A client of mine was convinced that she had lung cancer by using the muscle testing. Every time she tested 'Do I have lung cancer?' her body would react with a 'Yes' response. She became very stressed because she'd convinced herself even before testing that she had lung cancer. This shows the importance of being properly trained to understand your body's responses.

Here is a list of some basic things you can test through:

1. Is it about my (or insert emotion applicable) today?
2. Would my body benefit from eating (insert applicable type of food) now?
3. Will my body benefit from (insert applicable exercise) now?
4. Do I need to take my flower essence now?
5. Do I need to set a personal goal / affirmation?
6. Do I need to focus on the homework I have been given from my Kinesiologist?

Have fun with it, but remember that Kinesiology does not attempt to keep people away from doctors, medicine, surgery or the skills of any health professional they may need. Kinesiology focuses on unresolved stress reactions and uses techniques intended to assist the body's natural healing process.

I believe that our bodies have an innate healing energy and at all times do the best they can to heal themselves, yet at times through poor diet choices, poor physical choices, negative thought patterns, lack of belief, etc., we do not support this healing. Kinesiology can help our bodies into a better position to allow for this healing energy to flow through every cell within our bodies.

On a subconscious intuitive level our bodies know what we need to do to facilitate healing. However, in our busy lives we do not listen or get in tune with our bodies. Through Kinesiology we are able to tap into our body on a subconscious level to hear what our body needs to live in a balanced state. When our bodies are not in a balanced state our health will suffer, we will feel emotional and feel low in energy. By listening to our bodies we are able to heal our bodies from the inside out, starting at the root cause.

Unfortunately, we often do not even know what or how our everyday choices are affecting our mind and body. Yet every choice we make about what we think, feel, eat, act, react or behave are affecting our whole body, on both a conscious and subconscious level. It is these everyday choices that we need to alter to enable us to live a life filled with happiness and good health. Kinesiology becomes a tool to enable us to determine and address these choices and empower us to make choices that will support our whole body – physical, emotional, nutritional and spiritual.

trauma therapist

Sacred Harmony

Mary Jo Mc Veigh

Why integration of spirit, mind and body creates and maintains health.

Scríobhaim an chaibidil seo chun onóir a thabhairt do mo shinsearacht Cheilteach Éireannach. Tá meon s'acu i m'aigne, i mo chroí agus i mo spiorad. Tugaim mo ghrá gan deireadh agus mo bhuíochas do mo shinsir.

I write this chapter in honour of my Celtic Irish ancestry, whose ways are still deep within my spirit, mind and body. My never-ending love and deep gratitude always.

In my thirty years as a social worker and trauma therapist I have noticed that there is constant movement into what is clinically in vogue. As fads must, the 'new designer' theory or technique renders the previous wisdom as yesterday's style.

I have reflectively watched this jostling and, while I applaud it if it benefits clients, I have noticed that no matter what trend is in fashion there is a steadfast tendency to separate mind, body, and spirit.

My focus is not on any dogma related to either of these ways of being in the world. The reason why I emphasise this (and, indeed, my reason behind my desire to contribute to this book) is my belief in integration – not separation – as a means to living a healthy life.

Public health campaigns encourage physical health through (for example) regular exercise, good diet and avoiding the consumption of high levels of alcohol, drugs and tobacco. Mental health campaigns encourage healthy mind through brain training, relaxation or mindful practices.

There is also acknowledgment in these fields that there is a connection between a healthy body and a healthy mind. There appears to be scant attention given to the health of the spirit. It is my contention that this is due, not only to the separation I previously mentioned but, moreover, the association of the spirit with religion.

It is my contention that spirit is not a religious matter but a health matter and that integration of spirit, body and mind is the path to deep healing and a healthy life.

Seeking a Definition

In writing of spirit I am addressing the unphysical aspect of a person's existence, that essential part of them from which their animating life force flows.

Have you ever seen a luminosity that seems to abound from a person and has a quality beyond the physical? This translucent sparkle is the animating life force I speak of. The healthier it is the greater it shines.

Aspects of what I write will reach out differently to each of you. More importantly, the wisdom you gain will not be what I have written but what you will have heard in your own spirit as you read the words. Therefore, at intervals, I will invite you to take a pause from reading and listen to yourself.

I would also suggest you read this chapter in a place of quiet retreat, not the rattling carriage of a commuter train on the way to work. This way you are more likely to hear from yourself what it is you need to hear from the words on these pages.

There may also be times throughout this chapter that you say, 'Hold on a minute! What Mary Jo is writing about is not spirit but the physical,' and if I were sitting with you I would reply, 'That's correct'. There may be others times you may say, 'But those ideas apply to the mind,' and I would reply with a resounding, 'YES'. My entire contention about healthy spirit, healthy mind and healthy body is that the practices that keep you fully healthy on all these levels should not look too different in nature from each other.

A Call for a Return to Integration

I have watched people in my life – professional and personal – neglect the wellbeing of their spirit because they defined themselves as not religious or spiritual. And in this neglect I watched them suffer, as well as struggle to connect to a part of themselves that could have unlocked so much healing for their mind, body and spirit.

I have watched others who talked of the need for their spirit to be healthy but – because they did not define themselves as religious – were bereft of practices to call upon.

Moreover, we practise in a dogma of the clinical paradigm that separates – the body belongs to the medical world, the mind to the mental health world, and the spirit to the religious/

spiritual world. It would appear that despite a few intellectual forays into discussion, separation continues and diffusion of healing continues.

Despite this dominant discourse on what constitutes health intervention, I have had many adults seek conversation about healing their fractured mind *and* spirit.

At first their voice almost drops into a shameful hush, as if to speak too loudly means they will be 'caught out'. Sometimes they censor themselves, wary of judgement with, 'This may sound strange but …' and often they begin with a disclaimer as if to legitimise their own reality free of stereotyping with, 'I am not religious *but* …'

Despite this initial reticence, when I inquire about their desire to talk about healing their spirit they speak of 'a hunger', 'a yearning', or a 'longing' that therapy and medication alone cannot satisfy.

Harnessing Cultural Wisdom

In my search to find a clinical paradigm that does not separate and can meet the needs of my clients for conversation about spirit, I found many indigenous cultural healing practices that interconnected mind, body and spirit.

For many indigenous cultures, this living cultural context of healing was almost lost as colonisation and industrialisation took hold. We would be mistaken if we thought that all the practices are gone. Fortunately, there is a re-emergence of interest and academic inquiry into traditional cultural healing.

In my research on worldwide indigenous

healing I found strikingly similar beliefs and practices across these cultures and to my ancestry. This research gave me permission to reach back into the wisdom of my own culture, the Celtic Irish, to find a more integrated approach to my work.

Due to the diversity of the tribal groups, it would be more historically correct for me to refer to the Celtic Irish in multidimensional terms rather than as a monolithic culture. Because I have chosen wisdom from my cultural ancestry, not for annotated accuracy but as a wisdom that can be used in modern times, I will use the broad terms 'Celt' and 'Celtic Irish' to describe the ideas and practices that I was drawn to.

I will also not be extolling the virtues of all Celtic Irish healing practices, nor espousing a romantic notion of all of them. Neither will I be writing a comprehensive anthology.

What I have chosen to do instead is to open the treasure chest I found of both metaphoric and practical wisdom. It is my hope that upon considering the contents of this knowledge trove you will find something as precious for your clients as I have for mine.

Spirit in All Things

The Celtic Irish believed all things have a spirit, from a tree to a queen, from a rock to a king. They did not believe in animate and inanimate objects that would divide the world into the living and non-living.

For them, all things have life. This 'life' emanating from all things is what they defined as spirit. The spirit of all things is not bound up for them in religious or spiritual practice. It is within each and every person, animal, plant and natural object. That is not to say that spiritual practices did not emerge from these beliefs. Ireland of the ancient Celt was steeped in practices of worship to deities of nature and sacred rituals.

In this chapter I will be using that aspect of Celtic wisdom that acknowledges the spirit as of all of life and hence part of the identity of a person to look at an integrated approach to health.

Gerard Manly Hopkins, the Welsh poet, captures this concept so beautifully in a poem that I feel its first verse needs to be replicated:

> *As kingfishers catch fire, dragonflies draw flame;*
> *As tumbled over rim in roundy wells*
> *Stones ring; like each tucked string tells, each hung bells*
> *Bow swung finds tongue to fling out broad its name;*
> *Each mortal thing does one thing and the same:*
> *Deals out that being indoors each one dwells;*
> *Selves – goes itself; myself it speaks and spells,*
> *Crying What I do is me: for that I came.*

While Hopkins was a Jesuit priest and wrote in relatively modern times from his Catholic faith basis, his words echo this ancient belief of spirit, especially in the two lines, 'Each mortal thing does one thing and the same ... Crying what I do is me: for that I came'.

Regardless of professional status, economic measure, indeed societal recognition, by being ourselves we are being who we were called into existence to be. It is our spirit that holds the voice that heralds, *'This is who I am.'*

Our spirit does not demand that we earn more, or achieve more, become thinner or look younger. It demands nothing. The cry of 'What I do is me' is not about a job or a status in life, it is not about doing in the sense of action.

It is about the act of being yourself.

The spirit is healthy when you live your life from this authentic place. When you come to know that, there is a unique luminous sparkle that is all you.

Invitation to Pause

Consider what the cry of your existence is; what the essence of your spirit is.

Sickness of Body Originates in Sickness in Spirit

The Celts believed that physical sickness originates in the spirit world. While I honour the different realms of Celtic Irish wisdom, when I am working in a health context I use this aspect of my ancestral wisdom as a metaphor.

The spirit world I turn to is not Tír na nÓg, the

land of my spiritual companions, but the internal landscape of a person, the unique essence of who they are. It is my belief that physical and emotional illness not only arises in the body and mind of a person but can at times stem from a sickness of their spirit.

Over the years I have had the honour of being a participatory witness for people's healing as their therapist. Different interventions from the cognitive to the creative assisted in their rediscovery of a healthier self.

In exploring what set people free from their struggle, often they would talk not of their mind or body but of what helped their broken or damaged spirit.

One man spoke of being on a surfboard riding a wave: 'My spirit soared'; a young boy who stepped onto the stage in a school play: 'All dropped away and my soul was free'; and a woman, when she sang, said, 'I was at one with my spirit.'

The descriptions of these activities were not spoken in terms of mere physical pleasure or intellectual enjoyment. There is a different quality to it, a quality that enlivens and invigorates.

A quality of a spirit in health. It is therefore important for a healthy lifestyle that you engage in activities that enliven and invigorate the spirit, mind and body, and not focus exclusively on one over the other.

The Wisdom of the Spirit

When people talked to me about the spirit aspect of their being, they talked about a deeper self.

This deeper self seemed to have a wisdom that people tapped into to assist them with their healing. These conversations have taught me that there is an innate wisdom in each of our spirits as effective as the wisdom of the mind and it can help us on the path of healing.

For far too many people this wisdom is lost or not spoken about. How can we find something we are not told existed? Children are taught about physical health and prevention from a very young age – that is what underlies advice to clean teeth and eat vegetables. From playing with toys to formal learning in school, children's minds are kept healthy. The conversations and practice of a healthy spirit for children is less common. It is therefore no surprise that as adults, the access to this wisdom is either lost or is a struggle to retrieve. Yet, the yearning for connection to the spirit is not.

Conversations with Yourself

This wisdom can be gained through conversation – conversation with self and conversation with other. The wisdom of your spirit can be heard within the quiet moments of life; they cannot happen if we do not give time to this silent practice.

While I love and promote meditation and relaxation practices and have listened to the voice of my own spirit, these are not the practices I am exclusively referring to. The ability to listen to your spirit does not require rigorous discipline; it requires silence and a preparedness to listen.

Sitting in silence in your garden, watching a butterfly at play allows your spirit to be heard.

Moving around your home as you clean with no radio or television blaring provides the silence for you to hear your spirit. Going to your favourite spot by a river is the perfect environment for your spirit to be heard.

You will know the voice of your spirit because it is not like the noisy din of the chattering mind. It is gentle. It does not ask anything of you, it does not drag you into the past or hurtle you into the future.

It simply speaks and often a gentle *aha* moment happens and you know what to do to be in tune with yourself. Moreover, as you stay with your spirit, your mind starts to quieten and your body feels calm and health moves through all your systems.

Invitation to Pause

Think about moments in your life when you felt what it was like in the core of your being, what it is that takes your spirit and sets it free. Call to mind a silent place you can visit and book regular dates in your diary to go to that place.

Conversations with Other

In the Irish healing tradition, an *Anam Cara* was someone to whom you turned to seek guidance, counselling and support. In my native tongue, Irish, *Anam* means 'soul' and *Cara* means 'friend'.

When you seek counsel with them, your *Anam Cara* attends to all aspects of your being – physical, emotional, psychological and spiritual. The Irish believed this was a cherished connection in whose loving guidance your spirit was healed and your full potential released.

I think one woman's words sums it up when she wrote to me after we finished some work together: 'This means so much more than anyone knows. It is about what it feels like in my core, my spirit being taken and set free.'

Your *Anam Cara* was not a mystical oracle, and not all connection was imbued with lofty notions of purpose. Words of struggle, laughter at silliness, deep intellectual grappling, and simple instructions all were honoured and seen as equally important.

Surfing, singing, dancing, gardening and walking at dawn, are all activities of the healthy spirit and were all given a reverent place in the conversations with your *Anam Cara*.

You did not have to wait until you were struggling or sick to speak with your *Anam Cara*. It was as much a preventative relationship as it was a curative relationship.

If the belief that prevention is better than cure stretches all the way from the ancients into modernity then we need to consider how to live from the authenticity of our spirit and embrace it in our health plans.

Invitation to Pause

Who can you turn to for your spirit health check? What activities, ways of being, add lustre to your translucent sparkle?

Four Vital Elements of Healing

There are four interweaving elements in the cultural context of Celtic healing that particularly attracted me: Connection, Balance, Harmony and Sacred Ritual.

Connection: Self

When connection between mind, body and spirit is strong, all parts are strong and healthy. Health starts with the need to honour this connection and treat yourself as an integration of all these parts.

If there is disruption in one there is disruption in all. The solution is not only to bring health to each one but to engage in your own spirit-mind-body health plan as a preventive method.

Take, for example, the immune system. The immune system as the body's major defence organisation is not just compromised by physical attack. It is undermined by other forces.

The hormone secreted by the adrenal gland in situations of helplessness and hopelessness depress the immune system. It inhibits the synthesis of antibodies, reducing the number and inhibiting the activity of the T cells.

From this one example we can see that the health of the immune system does not rely on a physical approach only. Working with the Connection principle means it is vital to know what compromises your emotional life, what brings your spirit into despair, and engage in practices that maintain hope.

It is important if you find yourself in seemingly helpless or hopeless situations to find someone who can carry hope for you and who will support you as you find your way back from despair.

> **Invitation to Pause**
>
> Notice how you are fully connected to all parts of yourself. Make a commitment to yourself to do some small thing to keep this connection healthy.

Connection: Others

We humans are not separated from the spirit of all things. We are part of and belong to all things created. It was important for personal health in the Celtic world to have this healthy connection and to hold this connection with reverence. It is a connection of eternal belonging.

Living with healthy connection to all of life is more important now than it was in the times of my ancestors. We ignore this sacred connection of our spirit to the spirit of all of life at our own peril. In looking after others – human and animal, land and water – we will thrive. In taking care of this beautiful planet on which we live, we will thrive. Each of us has a unique connection to people, place and the great gifts of nature. We do not have to be part of organised environmental movement to keep this connection and ourselves alive and healthy.

> **Invitation to Pause**
>
> Notice what connection to the spirit of all things that you have. Make a commitment to yourself and this connection to do some small thing to keep this connection healthy.

Balance

The Celtic Irish healers encouraged the seeking of balance to maintain health. This balance was seen as internal to an individual person – a balance of mind, body and spirit.

The balance that was seen to be vital for health within the individual is also important in the relationship between the individual and all elements of their life. If one part of your life is unattended then the flow-on effects will be felt through the person's entire life and system.

> **Invitation to Pause**
>
> Do a balance health check and if you notice any places of imbalances in your life consider how to correct this.

Harmony

With balance comes harmony, that beautiful synchronism of life that brings you along in its flow. Life in harmony is when the congruency of all elements of your life forges together. You can have a harmonious life if you are living from the authentic core of your spirit, are connected to other people, hold dear your relationship with this living planet and all her inhabitants and creations.

Health is being in harmony but not just with one aspect of life. Health is when all aspects of who you are – your internal personal world and external connections – are in harmony.

> **Invitation to Pause**
>
> Do a harmony health check and if you notice any places of disharmony in your life consider how to correct this.

Sacred Ritual

Connection, balance, and harmony for health are not things to be taken for granted. There was a sacredness about them that the Irish Celts believed we needed to give praise and gratitude for. They embodied this in celebrations and sacred rituals.

Rituals are the customary procedures of life, not the domain of religious groups. All public health service delivery has its ritual – from the length and frequency of medical appointments to the formalities involved in a hospital admission.

So it is possible to have sacred ritual as an activity of honouring the connection, balance and harmony in your life without a religious bent. These rituals are not just an act of gratitude but also part of healthy spirit. We can build these rituals into the flow of daily life and turn to them as a health practice as much as we turn to the gym for fitness practice.

> **Invitation to Pause**
>
> Consider all you have in life and create your own rituals of acknowledgment and thanks. Think of the uniqueness of your spirit and devise your sacred rituals that keeps the vitality of your translucent sparkle glittering.

Beannacht

One of my favourite Celtic Irish sacred rituals was that of offering 'beannacht', translated to mean 'blessing'. In post-Christian times in Ireland, this was associated with religious blessings. Beannacht, however, has roots that are not connected to formal religious practice but in the ritual of invocation that is part of everyday life.

A beannacht was a ritual of words that honoured the spirit of all things and the eternal belonging of all of life. The person offering beannacht often invoked the gifts of the natural elements for themselves or others. People looked to the potential for healing within the words and the act of offering not just in the hoped for outcome as a results of reciting beannacht.

Parting Thoughts

As I come to the end of this chapter I now pause with you to think about what I have written. I have written from a place deep within my spirit, the only place I could write from when contributing to the ongoing conversation on preventive health. I have written not with the guile of thinking that the Irish way is the only way, but with the words that arose from my spirit. Therefore, my parting gift to you is in the tradition of the sacred ritual of innovation and my hope that you can use something in this chapter to add to the lustre of your luminous sparkle.

May you live in sacred harmony with all that is around you.
May you always be in the companionship of your luminous sparkle.

May you allow the connection to the earth to teach you.
May you call upon the balance of the elements to guide you.
May you harness the harmony of the universe to heal you.

May you live in sacred harmony with all that is and around you.
May you always be in the companionship of your luminous sparkle.

marketing strategist

Challenging Your Mind for Greatness

Samantha Jansen

'The space and time in your innermost dominant thought determines your outer-most tangible reality.'

– Dr John Demartini

Most people have gone through some kind of life-changing situation at one time or another. You might know people who recently separated from their partner or are grieving the death of a loved one, or someone who is unemployed and can't a find a job, struggling financially, or challenged in some other way. You might be their emotional or financial support system. We hear these stories frequently.

Most situations usually have warning signs along the way. I like to call them 'traffic lights', like when the lights change from green to orange – we know it's time to hit the brakes and slow down. Similarly, I use it as an example to remind myself of being conscious of my day to day surroundings.

Sometimes, we notice these signs, but turn a blind eye. Then, boom! Suddenly, the whole situation is out of control.

Fact: We all know someone who has been or have been in these shoes ourselves. One way or another, we might be connected to these situations.

Action to Transformation: Accept your surroundings and acknowledge them. You can learn a lot if you give yourself the opportunity.

I still have moments where, for a split second, I freeze and think, *Okay, what is my next step?*

It's okay to have moments which scare you and challenge you. These moments help you grow and give you a sneak peek at what opportunities might lie ahead.

As I share my journey with you – which changed my belief system, mindset, and transformed my life in ways I couldn't imagine – I hope this chapter gives you clarity and a sense that *you can do this also!* These steps are designed to help you acknowledge your dark times, awaken your awareness, and find your *aha* moments.

Give yourself permission to uncover a way of thinking which can transform your life.

My Transformational Story

My partner kept telling me, 'We need to spend more time together as a couple, rather than you always just being mum to our daughter.' I was so self-absorbed being a mum, I forgot how to be Samantha, the fun, cool and spontaneous girl he loved. I needed to pay more attention to him. But I was struggling – struggling to juggle motherhood, full-time work, a partner and running a household. Plus, I was pregnant, too.

BOOM!

The tension and the resentment grew and we couldn't keep living in the same household. He moved out, wanting to live his life on his terms. I was now a single mum raising a newborn and three-year old.

Emotionally and physically I was challenged daily. I had to act strong. 'Cos that's what mums do, right? So I kept going and going for a few weeks, crying myself to sleep some nights and hoping for some sort of sign. I'm a Christian and believe in God. So my level of faith was intact and I believed I would get the clarity on my next move.

I was so wrong.

No matter how much I believed in God and was looking for clarity, I was still feeding my mind the wrong information, thinking, *I'm a single mum and my life is going to be a mess. How can I juggle it all?*

This lead to my subconscious processing sad and lonely thoughts too. I was emotionally down. I'd had moments in my life where I would be surrounded by people who cared about me so much, yet now I felt like I was sitting in a well with very little light and thinking, *How am I going to climb out?*

It was a dark time for me.

Action to Transformation

One morning I woke up and thought, *This nonsense is enough. I'm a driven women with great ambitions.* It was that simple thought that transformed my life and became my *aha* moment. I finally acknowledged my feelings, emotions and my strengths. This was me giving myself permission to wipe the slate clean and start on a different path.

Since then, I have spent countless hours looking back on my life and thinking, *Wow, I had that many signs, which I ignored.* My partner didn't just disappear; he expressed himself time and time again. However, the experience taught me lessons for which I will be eternally grateful.

If you are reading this and thinking, *Why would you be grateful for going on such a rollercoaster ride which caused so much pain?*, the truth is I learnt so much about myself, my strength and my weaknesses. I learned more lessons every time I looked at the situation from another angle.

A New Beginning from One *Aha* Moment

A simple acknowledgement that morning changed my life. It gave me confidence, motivation and inspired me to be something great. Since then I have been on a journey that has enriched my life.

I ask myself daily, 'What can I do better when I'm challenged? How do I lift myself up when I feel like crap and just want to sit and not be disturbed?'

The answers to these questions came over time. I focused my thoughts and physical energy on things that made me happy but also on things that inspired me.

Today, I'm a happier and more grateful person. I set some solid intentions that day which included planning my financial freedom and lifestyle. Those intentions were my driving force and kept my mind occupied.

Your Journey to Greatness

Have you paid attention to signs that frequently come up in your life? Maybe you are stressed about a situation at work or constantly feeling the pressure of juggling family life and a career. Reflect on the last week or last month – what has caused the tension and stress? Ask yourself questions, rather than blame the universe or point the finger. Day-to-day situations and conversations will always attract what you are feeling, thinking and doing.

I knew a lady who always complained about her day-to-day mishaps, constantly whinging on Facebook. She struggled to comprehend why things never got better. A few times I casually mentioned to her, 'Look at your beautiful child and family and be grateful, rather than focusing on being in debt and the health issues you've had.'

As humans, emotions take over. It's okay to cry. Feeling like crap and being confused is normal too. However, I'm a big believer you need to know when to dust off the dirt and pick yourself up. Lying in the dirt isn't the solution.

Give yourself permission to ride the emotions. It's the only way to completely feel it and the only way you will know what it's like to be free of it once you have transformed your life.

1. ACKNOWLEDGE your situation NOW!
2. ASK for HELP
3. BE willing to step outside your COMFORT ZONE.

If you can do these three steps at least three to four times a week, you will start to see some changes in your life.

Your current experiences are more than enough to transform your life as you move forward. These three steps will show you how to have more control of your thoughts and truly tap into your potential and uncover the genius within you.

The First Step
ACKNOWLEDGE Your Situation!
What is your day like today? Did it start off as a good day and then things started to go wrong?

A client once told me how their day got worse and worse and it all started with their morning toast getting burnt.

The truth is if your toast gets burnt, bin it, toast a new slice, and let the frustration go. The longer you hold onto the frustration, the longer you feel anxious and irritated.

It's the same with road rage; some drivers drive us nuts with their reckless ways. I must confess, I struggle to keep my cool sometimes – especially when my kids are in the car with me.

Over the years, though, I have learned and implemented that if someone makes me mad or cuts in front of me, I make fun of their stupidity, 'cos then I focus my energy on fun rather than anger.

In no way am I saying what they did was right – reckless driving is never to be applauded. But it's about controlling one's emotions.

Acknowledge your emotions and the situation and then look at it from a different angle.

The Second Step
ASK for Help
We all could do with people helping us and outsourcing some of our day to day duties. Could

a family member help mind the kids? Can your partner do the cooking? Can the older kids hang out the laundry? True? But do we ask for help?

If you knew me a few years ago, I would never ask for help. I was ashamed to ask for it. I had a perception in my head that I was expected to be a strong, tough, resilient woman. But deep down I was in pain from being mentally, physically and emotionally exhausted.

I felt like I was a one-woman-circus, juggling motherhood, being a daughter, a partner, a sister, a friend, a colleague and a business owner.

The moment I decided to change my life, I started to ask for help.

I felt so much better, just having a few people help me with simple tasks. It gave me more time to focus on doing things which inspired me.

These were the stepping stones for me to become better as a person and achieve all I wanted and create my ideal lifestyle.

The Third Step
BE willing to step outside your COMFORT ZONE
After acknowledging your situation and seeking help to transform your life, the final stage and most important step is taking action.

Stepping outside your comfort zone is hard work. I have been there and done that.

Was it easy? Hell no!

Was it worth it? YES, YES, YES – every moment and sacrifice I made lead me to a better me.

I struggled at times; I had this weird feeling in my stomach, like knots tightening. But I kept pushing through.

The outcome was amazing. I remember what some of those days felt like; I was scared and anxious. I had young kids counting on me. Was I making the right decisions? It took hard work and conditioning my mind to keep going. Some days were harder, especially when people questioned me.

What did I decide to do? I couldn't physically juggle working fulltime in the city, running back and forth with two kids under the age of four. So I decided to quit my job and start a business using my skills and knowledge.

Over time I learned to ignore and not worry about what people said and decided not to take advice from people who didn't have any experience on the situation.

You would not ask a financial planner about fixing a broken car, so why take advice from someone with no experience in that situation?

People have a tendency to always have some sort of advice. Unless they have walked the talk, I don't believe they have what it takes to advise an individual. I still give them an opportunity to express themselves, I like to explore their suggestions and think about the problem from another angle. Thereafter, I make my own decision.

Have you ever experienced a little voice in your head debating why a decision might be good or bad? That's your ego. At that stage you know it's time to take control of your mind and make a decision.

Challenge yourself, take control, and start moving in the right direction.

Follow your gut feeling – nine times out of ten your instinct is right.

Does it follow comfort and known territory or does it advocate the unknown path?
I think you know what the answer is.

> ### Challenge Yourself
> I suggest challenging yourself and your mind. This will take some practice.
>
> Listed below are three simple steps to practise daily (at least 5 – 6 times a week):
>
> 1. Spend about 5 – 10 minutes in absolute silence recalling all the conversations you had in a day.
> 2. Think about what you said. Did you motivate or inspire the people you spoke to? Did you complain about a situation or a person?
> 3. Now ask yourself, 'If I could relive that moment, would I respond differently?'
>
> Eight out of ten times, you would respond differently to that situation if you were given a second chance. We get so caught up in the moment, we don't realise the impact we've caused by saying positive or negative things.

Click It, Change It

Over the years I have discovered a few things which help me get through tough moments when decisions need to be made and I need self control.

I'm not perfect; I still have more to learn and experience. I'm just aware of my surroundings and it takes me only about three to five minutes to realise I need to snap out of a negative situation or change the topic of conversation when I'm listening to negativity.

You might be feeling burnt out, exhausted from life's 9 – 5 rat race, feeling unloved and unappreciated, and know you want to make a difference and take control because deep within you there is a fire burning.

STOP self-sabotaging yourself. You are not meant to be living life on other people's terms. You have done enough for others and loved ones.

This is your moment to take control!

'Flick the switch from I Can NOT to I WILL and give yourself the opportunity to change your lifestyle. The power is within you.'

– Samantha Jansen

I learned to acknowledge everything I'm feeling. The more I acknowledge, the better it felt.

It's okay to be scared and freaked out sometimes. It's okay to not have all the answers. Yet it's important for your development to have the ability to acknowledge you are right where you are meant to be and to give yourself a pat on the back and say, 'I have come a long way. I can do this'.

I have met so many people and worked with quite a few who don't have a lot of support. When they start to make these changes and start to visualise a better lifestyle and dream of great things, they start to understand they are their own best friend.

Sometimes this can cause individuals to feel undervalued. I strongly recommend positioning yourself with people who value and believe in similar things as you.

As I have grown, my social circle has changed. I love socialising with my friends and family – some more than others due to stimulating conversations we have. They all impact my life one way or another and I'm grateful for each one of them. I don't expect everyone to understand and be on the same page as me. We are all different. Since I started this journey, I needed like-minded people so I joined various networks and attend events.

Today, I'm actively a part of multiple networks and business communities. This gives me opportunities to learn and improve myself, but also implement techniques which would benefit my clients.

What is your situation right now?

Are you aware of your surroundings?

Let's challenge your mind and break through limiting beliefs.

Breakthrough to Greatness

Fact – you are like the five people around you!

Since breaking through and giving myself an opportunity to create a life I love, I have noticed the people I attract are much more like me. Since I made a conscious decision I was going to change my life, some of my friends and family drifted away. We still speak, but we are no longer as close as we used to be. This made way for new people to come into my life. These people support me, help me and hold me accountable.

If you look at your immediate circle of family or friends, they will have similar interests to you. That's why you find it so easy to get along and they are within your tight circle.

If you can take one thing from reading this chapter, let it be that you acknowledge that you are right where you are meant to be. Nothing happens by chance. Everything is by something we did to trigger that situation or outcome. Either subconsciously we kept saying, 'It's not going to happen', or 'It's going to work out well.'

Once you acknowledge and start being grateful for everything you have, you will start to see a shift happening.

Over the years I have noticed people who complain will always complain. They thrive on it. People who are complacent will just keep going and the next group, The Achievers (they have BIG dreams – I hope you are in this one), they believe in themselves and acknowledge their self-worth.

Are you ready to transition and improve your life? To break through situations which are currently holding you back? I truly believe you have the power to do it. It's within you. I consult people who thought they couldn't move forward. They believe they are not worthy or don't know how. The truth is your mind is a powerful machine. You just need to give it a jump start and your thoughts will be flooded with knowledge and ideas. I'm not a counsellor or physiologist; I'm a mum, a partner, a daughter, a sister, a friend, a colleague, a mentor, a coach and a business owner. Everything I share with you is from my own journey. I experienced it, and learnt and implemented things to transform my life.

I transitioned from being a satisfied individual to acknowledging I can have everything I want and dream. It doesn't matter what it might be. The moment I started changing my mindset and my way of thinking, I reprogrammed my subconscious to think of creating success in my life. My success is up to me and only me. I can sabotage it, settle for second best, or do something to change my life.

We all have a choice in life. People often want to change because they are sick of feeling drained, burnt out and caught between what they want and what they have. However, most people are too scared to go outside their comfort zone. Those who are willing to step into the unknown and dare to challenge themselves have a higher chance of success. Why? Because they are willing to take action to change their situation.

When I made a decision to change, it didn't happen overnight. It took months and months. I gave myself daily goals. Some were simpler than others. The key was taking steps that were different to my usual lifestyle. Acknowledging I can change the small habits, talking less and listening more to what was around me and be willing to examine myself and think, *Why did I do that?* or *Why did I say that?* gave me the confidence, inspiration and motivation to believe I could accomplish my goal to create my ideal life and business.

> 'We can achieve greatness, if we believe in it – it's within us!'
>
> – Samantha Jansen

The key to breaking through tough times was changing my mindset – giving myself some me-time to reflect and recharge, reading books on personal development and being grateful for every situation – the good and the bad (trust me, the bad ones teach you too).

Transforming your life begins with you setting your intentions. Why not start right now? Do not worry about the drama and tension in your life. Find one thing and focus on that and then focus on two things and keep moving along. As time goes on, you will have moments where your thoughts start to become clearer as your mind has been subconsciously programmed to think of the positive activities rather than the negatives.

Those who challenge their minds for greatness will always succeed. Their determination is strong and they will push themselves, be open to be mentored and look for ways to improve themselves.

Think of athletes competing for a spot in the Olympics. They have a coach helping them train every single day for months and even years, then the athletes are pitted against each other, and the best of the best make it to the top. Individuals who make it to the Olympics have trained, made sacrifices and learnt techniques to get the best out of themselves along the way. Their determination and commitment to succeed is one of their highest values.

What do you want for your future? Remember, you hold the key and you have the power to achieve greatness. I hope you tap into the power within you and achieve greatness and success in everything you do.

art psychotherapist

The Art of a Healthy Mind

Isolde Martin

Keeping a healthy mind – yes, that is indeed of importance for an art psychotherapist, or any psychotherapist for that matter. Without it, therapeutic effectiveness would be compromised in various ways and a therapist might not last a professional lifetime.

I do think that the basis for keeping a balanced, sound mindset in this profession is similar to other so-called 'helping' professions. After all, we are human beings and are dealing with human beings.

In my experience, basic preparation for art therapeutic work started during the last two semesters in graduate school. This was, in my mind, a first line of defence. Perhaps one could also see it as a means of avoiding disequilibrium of our minds. We were watched during 'experiential' sessions, or when we exercised therapeutic work using each other as subjects. Personal problems would surface and thus could be dealt with. If nothing else, we simply had to face our own issues – issues that might affect our emotional suitability as an art therapist. We needed to face ourselves and be aware of our trouble spots in order to compensate or avoid problems later on.

This process continued and intensified during our internship. Of course, all of us had to go through our own therapy properly before we could attempt to work with our clientele. Armed with understanding our own psychological make up as much as possible, we had a good chance to avoid a troubled mind, or, if necessary, know how to deal with it.

In order to be able to do that we also were prepared to accept that we are not perfect and thus were open about our own shortcomings, rather than suppress or deny them.

Of course, it follows as a very important tool that we recognise the symptoms when our own psychological make up or our own past experiences threaten to surface and interfere.

Moreover, we needed to be comfortable with and still like our own person as a whole and the way we are. That, in a society that values perfection and does not take kindly to failure, was not an easy learning process. But it was necessary for confidence and inner strength.

In terms of personal trouble spots preparing the way for a mind in disharmony there is another important and often debated issue. Therapists deal with emotional problems every day, all day. Many clients have extremely painful, breathtakingly bad life stories.

In order for the therapist to keep being objective it is necessary to let empathy happen but to avoid suffering with the client. The latter is, for one, possibly counterproductive to the therapeutic goal. But, more importantly, if the therapist cannot balance empathy with co-suffering it is a sure way for her to experience burn out. Thus it is imperative to keep objectivity to stay balanced and keep a healthy mind.

Of course, there are also specific and highly effective tools to keep a healthy mind in a world that deals with the opposite, a troubled mind.

The following goes for all of us, the everyday person, a client (or patient as some would have it) and professional alike – we are all just people. The same issues make us tick; the same things frighten or please us. And for all of us the best line of defence is prevention.

Let's not wait until things have grown unbearable.

Our modern life is stressful all by itself. Thus, first we need to strengthen what we have on a regular basis, which means to practice mindfulness for one thing. People have various methods to do that. The most frequently mentioned and recommended method is mediation. But many ways can lead to Rome.

There are studies over studies that have investigated the usefulness and effectiveness of physical activities to reduce stress. The results are very much in favour of balancing a stressed person. Interestingly, any sport, be it walking or training seriously for a championship, particularly addresses psychological stress. The slogan would be: *Get out of your mind and into your body.*

For some of us it is greatly soothing and healing to change environment for just an hour, or a day, or a week. This is quite important. It is called 'taking a break'. That could mean we visit a theatre performance tonight, or we go outdoors and walk by a forest, a lake, or a mountain, we listen to the birds, and breathe fresh air, or we take a lengthier vacation elsewhere.

The idea is to get away from routine.

This should give us a chance to break an

unhealthy cycle. I used to have a colleague who went for a massage every Friday almost without fail. It worked for her.

This brings me to another point in preventing and reducing a troubled mind. Not all methods work for all people. We are individuals. It is necessary to find out what suits a given person best, what leaves us with a good feeling, and what takes a load off our minds.

What has a liberating effect on our mind and thus on our problems?

Such a change of routine, big or small (such as going dancing for the evening), has the potential to see our stressors or problem in a different light and from a different angle. Suddenly, the things that held us down seem solvable.

This all might sound a bit banal and matter of course. Well, perhaps, but it works very well. It keeps us centred and helps us to keep our objectivity with regards to clients or personal problems or anxieties which we all have at times. It can ease a stressed mind back into calm and peaceful waters.

All of the above is fine but not exhaustive. There is another issue that is absolutely necessary to reduce the incident of a stressed mindset. Clear boundaries have to be set and kept between work and private life.

We are human beings with limited energy and a need for freedom from obligations and challenges for a certain time period. For instance, it is advisable to limit us to taking only specific calls rather than being available all the time. This decision alone is comfort for our minds.

This is not just for an art therapist but for all of us. None of us are perfect, nor do we need to be. But that kind of thinking is very prevalent in this age and time. The result is a nearly permanent overload on our minds. The cure is a change in philosophy and then a reasonable reduction of stress. That might mean that it is necessary to keep friends, acquaintances, or colleagues and bosses, outside of our newly established boundaries.

Turning off our computers and mobile phones can work wonders for our mind. It means the freedom of letting our minds wander to more desired issues. The German people have a neat but potent slogan for recovering stability for our minds by 'getting away from it all':

Let your soul swing in the wind.

There is, of course, one obvious method and medium for art therapists which we use almost spontaneously and as a matter of course. You guessed it! We engage in artistic activities: paint, draw, sketch, model with clay, play in the sand, make music, compose poetry, write what is on your chattering mind.

This is for all of us to employ. It does not matter how well you can paint or write. You are doing this exclusively for yourself, not for anybody else. In practical terms, what is an easily available and effective tool to centre our troubled minds is to keep a journal – a painted, illustrated journal, needless to say.

And if the images that emerge are resisting understanding and interpretation, we paint some more. But then, just jotting down the things that burn on our mind and soul can have the lifting, liberating effect from trouble. Paper is patient and does not criticize or judge us.

Writing also makes us think about our problems in order to formulate sentences. That gives objectivity and rationality as chance. It can put issues into perspective. When writing we always also talk to ourselves. As we get our troubling thoughts out of our mind and onto paper, we often feel a load lift.

So listen to yourself.

It does not always feel good to face our problems but it should feel good at the end. For people who are hesitant or even frightened to see your problems in front of you, it might be advisable to seek the help of a therapist. Don't be bashful, this is what they are there for.

Many of us are engaged in an artistic process in an ongoing fashion. That makes us deal with the happenings of the day. There is the painting on the easel waiting for us when we have spare time. There is the sketchbook in the bag accompanying some all the time.

Others carry a camera with them to catch and fix what their artist's eyes are pointing out. After all, there is a reason for choosing the images we take pictures of. All these activities have the great potential to take us away from an overloaded mind. But better yet, they help us to keep future stresses at bay.

These methods of stress management and reduction are for every person with a bothered, tired mindset. These are very effective tools to help us, clients, patients and everyday people come back to a calm and healthy mind. If you are not sure how to start then do just that. Start with the one activity that looks easiest to you, raises the least anxiety (as it does with some people) and leaves you with an uplifted feeling at the end.

Speaking about getting 'it' out: One spontaneous and sometimes ad hoc method to clear our mind is our colleagues and friends. They are there right after a session, after a day. They have felt like me, you, us before and have understanding, empathy, and advice if need be.

And they are, for the most part, good, patient listeners, which sometimes is all it takes. I once had a colleague coming out of her office holding her forehead and exclaiming, 'I am losing it! I am losing it!' Baffled, we stood there watching her until one of us asked the obvious.

'What are you losing?'

'I am losing my mind!'

Well, I doubted that, along with my colleagues. 'Come, we have a staff meeting now. Let's talk about it.'

And she did and we listened. She was all right after that. Talking to friends can be a powerful tool as a mind healer if you are able to be open and honest. Find another human being, a friend, an acquaintance, a family member, or any significant other that you trust and who's opinion you value.

I once got my own dose of such kindness, empathy, and help for my troubled mind. My mother had passed away. I had been with her the last weeks of her life, and watched her die. I drew a grave with a wreath on it and my mother's name and dates on the tombstone. This I sent to my colleagues. After my return to work there came the first group therapy session I needed to attend.

'Can you handle it if the issue of death and dying comes up?' I was asked.

Yes, now I could. I was not alone but rather had support from my colleagues.

Of course, we don't engage in all of those methods to keep a healthy mind in our activities all the time. But mental stress is a part of life for all of us.

With the right regularly applied exercises, we can reduce the impact on our minds and keep it on a healthier level to begin with. The magic word is prophylaxis.

This, of course, is not always possible. Over time, what works best for a given person will crystallize out of all the methods available. One just has to try them out. At the end, it is important to become aware and learn the personal signs of stress and notice them approaching. Then one can immediately reach for the paint brush.

Try this as an exercise for a calmer mind:

Please keep in mind that it does not matter whether you 'can draw' or you feel you cannot. Anybody can hold a pen, a crayon, or a paint brush and draw. You do this for yourself only, not for anybody else. Only you have to like it, nobody else.

Directive

With whatever art materials you like to use, draw or paint a place for yourself that you would like to be in.

It can be any place – real, or created out of your imagination and wishes. And if you insist you cannot draw, take a pair of scissors and old magazines and cut out pictures. Make a collage from them as long as it becomes a place you would like to be in.

For a special touch draw yourself into your place. Yes, stick figures are also okay. If you say this represents you, then it is you. No criticism!

Directive

In an abstract way, draw a characteristic of yours that you like.

Again, don't worry about your artistic skills. You do this by yourself and for yourself.

Happy painting and enjoy!
Take good care of yourself.

social entrepreneur

Trust and Respect

Galen Dean Loven

Very seldom are we challenged to look at these two very important, value-laden words – 'trust' and 'respect' – in regards to mental health and well being.

Most certainly we seldom look at them in concert. The reason they are packaged together in this undertaking is that both words are frequently misused, causing confusion and distancing from personal responsibility and accountability.

Before discussing how these two words are often closely connected, I will examine them individually.

Trust
Have you ever heard, or used, either of these phrases ...?

'I just want to trust you'
or
'How do I know I can trust you'?

What is meant by these statements?

In most relationships the speaker is saying, 'I want you to take care of me.' Or, 'I want to know you will look after me.'

Thus trust gets mixed in with a lot of relationship issues, victim positioning, and guilt. This does an excellent job of disturbing our mental balance as our inner being hears one word (trust), yet must respond to an entirely different set of expectations and meanings.

It is helpful to understand what 'trust' really means. Many definitions use some form of predictability in describing 'trust', 'trusting' or 'trustworthy'.

Many definitions also invoke societal values, such as caring for another's well being. It becomes quite confusing trying to sort out all of these qualitative statements.

Let's reduce trust to its most basic element:

The ability to predict a person's behaviour in a given set of conditions.

This strictly quantitative definition removes a lot of the value-laden elements normally associated with trust. It allows a clear test bed for determining trust, and trustworthiness.

For example, you know someone who is a violent drunk. You can predict that when drunk, that person will be violent.

In other words, you can *trust* that person to be violent when drunk. If that person is consistently violent when drunk, then s/he is trustworthy to be a violent drunk.

In the same vein, that person may also be a highly reliable worker, never missing a day of work, regardless of how ill (or hung over). You can predict that this person will show up for work in a timely manner. You can trust this person to be on time for their job.

Continuing, it is possible that this person is

quite unpredictable when keeping non work-related appointments, sometimes being on time, sometimes late, sometimes not showing up at all. All you can predict is unreliability with respect to personal meetings or appointments. You can *trust* this person to be unpredictable.

Perhaps the most striking aspect of trust is that it does not include hope. Hope is an expression of desire, which is often blended in with the 'confusing' use of trust, such as 'Can I trust you?' meaning, 'Will you take care of me?' Trusting is unemotional expectation based upon experience.

I have just introduced the element of experience. Logically it is not possible to predict a person's behaviour in a given set of conditions unless you have observed (or have reliable information on) that person's behaviour in similar conditions. Trust is earned, or garnered through experience.

One reason for the relationship history questions in a new relationship is the need to determine predictable behaviour. For example, 'You acted in such-and-such a way in your last relationship(s), so I can predict you will be that way with me.'

While this may in fact be true, it limits the person being interviewed to past behaviours, providing absolutely no opportunity or scope for new ones.

Bringing expectations based upon old experiences into new relationships makes it almost impossible for a person to adopt new, healthier behaviours, or for the person in the new relationship to be 'trusted' for who and what they are at the moment.

Perhaps you have experienced this frustration yourself when you have solved a behavioural glitch (like co-dependence), yet find yourself constantly defending the 'new' you. It is not fair, nor healthy, to be trapped like this.

The other side of this definition of trust is that once someone has acted unpredictably it is no longer possible to rely on the previous predictable behaviour.

This means that once trust has been broken it is impossible to recover due to the previous unpredictable act, because it could always happen again.

In a relationship, the healthiest way to develop trust is to work from the experiences you have with the person you are involved with, rather than the experiences they have had with others. This is particularly important as no two relationships are ever the same.

On a similar note, it is important to understand your own behaviours in given conditions or circumstances. If you are changing, then you must allow for those changes when making those harsh self-evaluations.

You must also be discerning and diligent to ensure that you isolate each type of behaviours you examine for trustworthiness.

It is entirely possible, and in fact probably so, that the degree of trustworthiness will vary according to the particular behaviour and circumstances.

Respect

How often have we said, or heard someone say, 'I just want some respect!'?

Respect: (http://dictionary.reference.com/browse/respect)

1. esteem for or a sense of the worth or excellence of a person; a personal quality or ability, or something considered as a manifestation of a personal quality or ability.
2. deference to a right, privilege, privileged position, or someone or something considered to have certain rights or privileges; proper acceptance or courtesy; acknowledgment.

While we often believe that the second definition is the one referred to in that exclamation, more frequently the implied meaning is the first one. This means that we feel a lack of acknowledgement or appreciation rather than a lack of position recognition. Certainly when we use the word when referring to others, such as 'I have no respect for him/her', we mean that we have no positive regard for that person.

Genuine respect can only be earned. The respect we often seek for ourselves is for our personal qualities more than we seek recognition for those things we know or do. So important is the need for appreciation of ourselves, that we often DO things for others hoping that they will respect us for what we have done for them. This often results in the opposite reaction, especially when charity, enabling, or co-dependency is involved.

The question is how can we earn respect?

The answer is simple to state, very hard to do.

To earn the respect of others we must respect ourselves.

While our first response might be, 'Of course I respect myself', a more thoughtful consideration would most likely reveal that we are looking for the respect granted from others to help us feel better ourselves (giving us self-respect). Unfortunately, it does not work that way.

Self-deception comes from many sources, many of which were developed when we were young, forcing ourselves to conform to what we were told we had to be or do to be acceptable, cared for, or loved. This pattern is very hard to break, yet is critical if we are to become resonant with ourselves, thus gaining that important self-respect.

This is a good time to take a more thorough look at the power of lies.

Our society is highly qualitative (and implied-meaning oriented) when it comes to the term 'lie'. For example, there are many types of lies such as:

- white lie
- black lie
- little lie
- big lie
- bald-faced lie
- unintentional lie
- lies of commission
- lies of omission
- mis-speak.

This list is by no means exhaustive, just illustrative of the extent of lying in our society. Of course, the most immediate question that comes to mind is, 'What is a lie?'

Webster's New Collegiate Dictionary, G. & C. Merriam Company, 1979 defines 'lie' as:

1. To make an untrue statement with intent to deceive
2. To create a false or misleading impression.'

There are two salient aspects to this definition:

1. the **intention** of deceit or misdirection (versus an unintentional act – a mistake)
2. the **effect** of creating an understanding of something that is not true (regardless of degree).

In other words, lying involves a deliberate act to sabotage another's perception about a given situation.

This raises the question of whether or not it is possible to 'lie to oneself' as it may be assumed that the individual attempting to deceive his/herself would also be aware of the attempt. For the moment, to avoid a detraction into metaphysics, we will concern ourselves with situations involving two or more parties.

What happens when a lie is perpetrated?

The person on whom the deception is practised becomes disadvantaged in that s/he receives a distorted sense of what is going on.

Whether or not the deception is ultimately harmful depends upon the reliance of the deceived on the deception, and the nature of the lie relative to other activities.

Regardless, once the deception is revealed the deceived will lose at least some confidence in the other.

The real harm in lying comes to the liar. The reason for this is in the nature of deception. To create a lie, an individual must step outside of reality.

Once this is done, the lie becomes a new reality. It requires time and energy to maintain. The longer a lie persists, the more time and energy it takes to maintain.

Clearly the lie begins to assume a life of its own. It grows in strength and power over time and usage. The perpetrator becomes trapped by the lie. Essentially, the life of the liar will be altered by the lie.

In addition to the effort it requires to sustain a lie, there are the risk factors associated with avoiding having the lie exposed, and the emotional and psychic energy required to maintain a sense of equilibrium.

While it may seem that the extent of a lie affects its ability to control a life, it is not necessarily so. Life is causal.

We cannot predict the effects of a given action as it ripples through our lives. Thus, we cannot truly predict what effects creating a lie might have.

So what happens when a lie is told?

The recipient does not receive useful information that is meaningful, and the deceiver wastes energy in protecting the falsehood.

Under such circumstances it is difficult to imagine a scenario in which telling a lie would be appropriate or constructive.

Thus, the lies we tell about ourselves, those we use to make ourselves conforming to the expectations of others, are the most damaging to ourselves.

If we are lying to ourselves, we know this at some core level or deeper consciousness. When we do so, we cannot respect ourselves because we know that we are not truthful.

A real trap exists because we do not perceive how we can undo our history of untruthfulness. The fear is that we will be treated worse than we are, or that we will be loved less, or that something really bad would happen.

Sadly, the worst things that we fear might happen probably already *are* happening because of our own lack of respect and truthfulness.

While we usually know when we are misrepresenting or lying to others, it is often difficult to know when we are lying to ourselves. As a rule, creative and/or intelligent people are much better at self-deception than others.

This is because they are more ingenious at spinning authentic-seeming weaves and stories. The inner self is aware of the lack of truthfulness. The internal conflict results in many physical manifestations of dis-ease, and naturally enough, the lack of self-respect.

How do we know when we are lying to ourselves?

It is perhaps not very strange that many of the symptoms of self-deception are associated with, or diagnosed as other forms of illness or dis-ease.

Cautioning that there are no absolutes, and that there are more than one cause for many illnesses, the following shortlists can be good indications that you are not in accord with your true, or core, self (often called self-resonance):

- psoriasis
- asthma
- accidents causing pain or injury
- ulcers and digestive problems.

Some of the more psychological symptoms can be:

- panic attacks
- depression
- suicidal tendencies
- uncontrollable anger and rages
- use of affirmations.

What are some of the things about which we deceive ourselves?

- we have no choices
- we are powerless
- we are victims
- we are being truthful
- we are spiritual
- that we are responsible for the happiness of others
- that we are worth-less.

Unfortunately, most of these self-deceptions were learned at a very early age. We were trained that we had to conform to expectations if we wanted to be fed, clothed, or loved. We had to dis-engage from our core self, adapt and change, becoming what those who had control over our lives decided was acceptable.

It is true that when we are infants, and in many degrees, until we are adults, we are dependent upon others for our survival. The lessons of helpless-ness and powerless-ness, coupled with that great controller – guilt – that we learn are then deeply ingrained in our psyche.

The confrontation between who we are as core individuals, and what we have become, is postponed. We have built a pattern of self-deception and lying about ourselves that can be very difficult to overcome.

Some of us never have to meet this challenge. We have become comfortable in the roles we were given. Some of us, however, are not comfortable, developing some of the symptoms listed earlier. We are the ones who must confront ourselves and determine ways to gain self-respect and truthfulness.

One of the hardest things to do is overcome habits – impediments, or barriers to healthier, more truthful, behaviours.

Guilt

We are a judgmental by nature. When we decide to stop one behaviour in favour of another we naturally put that negative value on the old one saying it was 'bad' and that is why we have to stop doing it.

Perceived loss of investment

A natural result of assuming a new behaviour is the condemnation we place on what we were doing.

In other words, we look at ourselves as stupid, weak, ignorant, or worse yet, bad, because we had been acting in way that is neither comfortable nor desirable. We self-damn ourselves, and part of us does not want to 'give up' all that time and energy we've invested in our past behaviours.

The phrase, 'If I knew then what I know now, I never would have done this' should be embraced at this time. Because you do know better now, this is the time to act differently.

Self-damnation makes it harder to get past the old behaviour or thought.

How would you know if you were affected by these issues?

The first clue should be words or phrases that you use when discussing the no longer desired behaviour(s).

Examples are ...

- 'How could I have been so stupid?'
- 'I can't believe I did that.'
- 'S/he wasn't really a bad person. I must have done things to make him/her hurt me.'
- 'What does this say about all of those years I spent doing ...?'

Another clue is whether or not reading this makes you uncomfortable. If it does, the odds are pretty good that you are responding to a trigger about some fear or subconscious resistance to change.

How insidious is this programming?

A good friend of mine continues to stay firmly routed in old, destructive behaviours with her son (now in his thirties) because of guilt she has concerning his upbringing.

It is amazing to watch them. Neither are happy with the relationship yet both continue to perpetrate the dance of dis-ease and unhealthy patterns. Her anguish and his anger are exceeded only by the vortex of nervous energy they generate when together.

What works?
Look at the words you use
A good process is to look at what kind of words you use when attempting new patterns. Many of the mantras and affirmations carry potent messages of blame and judgement about the old behaviours.

For example, instead of just replacing 'I have to fight for my rights' with something else, first put the old one constructively away.

Instead try saying something like this, 'I have fought for my rights, now I have them.'

A little different spin on things but a big difference in internal perception.

Watch out for the phrase 'I am trying.'

This is a great word of avoidance. In the future whenever you hear that phrase (whether spoken by yourself or another) substitute the words, 'I am doing ....' or 'I am not doing ...'

Take a hard look at the veracity, or truthfulness, of those phrases in each particular situation. Chances are it will be a different viewpoint.

Then begin using only those two phrases for yourself when discussing your behaviours and what you wish to achieve. The clarity of 'do or not doing' will be a great aid in going forward.

Look at the behaviours you want
What is it that you want to do in your actions? Instead of just saying 'I need to be different', write down the behaviours and activities you wish to adopt. Think about what they are as opposed to the ones you wish to replace. Write those ones down as well. Examine the two lists side by side.

Now think about how you feel or felt when you were acting in the old manner.

Then think about how you would or do feel acting in the new manner.

What is different about those feelings?

Write those feeling down, both sets side by side.

The difference in emotional content is a pointer. It will lead you to what you are all about.

It is possible that you do not feel as 'good' in your new behaviours as you might think or wish.

You might even be resentful or bitter about the 'need' to act differently.

It is also possible that you feel better with the new behaviours. How is that better feeling? Is it more respectable, calmer, safer or is there a deeper feeling involved?

These feelings, and how you react to them, are extremely important for the next step of the process – moving towards truthfulness and self-respect.

Affirmations

Another way to stay stuck in place is the use of what is commonly known as 'positive affirmations'. The pitch behind affirmations is that if we continue to say something that we want, we will get it. For example, you want more money, so you put up affirmations saying, 'I am a millionaire!'

Everyday, often more than that, you look at this affirmation and repeat it with conviction. However, your subconscious knows that you are not a millionaire, and the reason you have this 'affirmation' is because you are not a millionaire. Your self sees the lie, and you are continuously re-enforcing (affirming) that you are not a millionaire.

An affirmation should be something that acknowledges what is good about you, not what is lacking. Every day most of us receive affirmations but never recognize them for what they are. They are usually simple things like:

- a smile from a cashier
- a child or friend giving you a hug
- a nice look from a stranger passing in the street
- a courteous driver
- a door held open for you
- a compliment at work.

Simply, things that happen daily without us appreciating them for what they are. To begin affirmations start a book, a special book. Write in it daily those things that happened to you that were affirming. It may be strange and awkward at first, and you may not have many entries. As time progresses, it becomes easier and there will be more entries each day. Not only will this help you feel better about yourself, you will be building the foundations of self-respect and a different, more powerful form of trust will enter your world. You will begin to trust yourself in a positive way.

We Come Now to the Heart of the Matter
Truthful versus Honest

How many people do we know (including ourselves) start a sentence with, 'Honestly ...'?

When I hear that, two thoughts run through my mind:

Oh, you weren't honest before? and
Why do you need to say 'honestly'?

One of the most insidious worms that eats away at our self-respect is a lack of truthfulness. Truthfulness is quite different from honesty. Truthfulness carries intention, honesty is a condition. For example, it is quite possible to be completely honest (as in not telling a direct lie) without being truthful. A quick test for this quality is to make an important statement about an important feeling in these two ways.

The first time beginning the sentence with, 'Honestly, I feel that ...'

The second time beginning the sentence with, 'Truthfully, I feel that ...'

Start your new life, the one based upon self-respect, and self-trust by using 'Truthfully' as your operative word. Place it in front of statements you make about yourself, and how you feel, including how you feel about others and the situation(s) you are in. Be certain to allow the heart intention to enter, and be certain to say these sentences out loud.

The two tools, truthfulness and genuine affirmations, will guide you well on the hard road to self-respect and trust. Yet, guide you they will. Truthfulness will help you lay to rest the old self-deceptions without a lot of anguish and guilt. Facts become just that – then knowing what you know now, you can and will act differently.

Real affirmations will help hold you to what is true about yourself. You will not need to define yourself by the standards of others. You will not need to spend thousands of dollars and countless days seeking answers and self worth that is already there, deep within, ready to surface into the bright light of truthfulness.

These tools are not guaranteed to bring you happiness. They will bring you peace and certainty and a knowledge of your self.

From there you can plot a course that is yours.

writer

Write For Your Life

Les Zigomanis

You wake up and, immediately, the day's responsibilities scramble through your head. If we could represent those responsibilities diagrammatically, they might look something like this:

            go to work
  take car for service   exercise
    see doctor   pay bill
          go shopping   cut lawn
      talk to bank   call Mum
        vacuum house fix window
   call plumber cook dinner
  take kids to school   answer emails
          check mail

From here, we'd begin to prioritise what we need to do, ranging from what needs attention urgently, to what can wait.

But the reality is that we don't think in words. We think in impulses, instincts, and emotions. If you want a cup of tea, you don't think, *I would like a cup of tea*. You have an impulse that correlates with tea. Then thought articulates that desire into language.

That's the way our brains work.

And they work well for matters that can be distilled precisely into language. A cup of tea is a cup of tea. There might be queries about how it's made (white, black, with sugar, with lemon, with honey, etc.) or the flavour of the tea (Breakfast Tea, Earl Grey, Chamomile, Green Tea, etc.), but your impulse will define exactly the course you're going to take.

Issues arise when we deal with things that are too complicated to distil. If you've ever lost somebody you loved, or had a relationship break up, or lost a job, you're dealing with an issue that hits you on every level – intellectually, emotionally, physically, and spiritually. If you were to articulate how you felt, you might simply say, 'I'm upset', but this hardly does the way you're feeling justice.

Every day, we deal with these sorts of issues. They mightn't be as weighty as the above examples, but they do happen. Think about the idiot who cuts you off in traffic. Or when a co-worker undervalues you. Or a friend says something hurtful. These sorts of things happen every day.

And how do we deal with them?

Usually, if we're that busy through our everyday lives – and most of us are – we spare these matters only peripheral attention. Sometimes, they demand that attention and spill over into our lives, affecting our everyday responsibilities. When they preoccupy us, that's when we fall into melancholy or depression.

Whatever the case, writing is something that can help.

Me

I've suffered depression, anxiety, OCD, and issues relating to these neuroses all my adult life, and much of my teenage life – at the time of writing this, over thirty years. Often, any (or all) of these things will pulse insidiously in the background – at best, like a coiled, poisonous snake whose very proximity destabilises you, and, at worst, like that damn snake has struck you.

On a baseline level, these neuroses influence my thought processes. Decisions aren't decisions – not the way everybody makes them. A trip somewhere, for example, isn't *just* a trip. My anxiety will explode it into a potential for disaster – car crash, plane crash, catastrophic health issues. The anxiety chatters away in my head, warning me of every worst-case scenario.

You'd think that it would be easy to disarm, but this is something people who've never experienced anxiety don't understand. It's not just nervousness or worry. It's not trepidation about doing something, like coming off the high diving board. It's debilitating and irrational fear. If you're phobic about anything (e.g. spiders, heights, blood), that's anxiety, only applied to everyday life, magnified, and kept thrust in your face every second of every minute of every hour of every day.

It's only in more recent years that I've come to understand innately how my own neuroses work, although that doesn't help dismantle them. We have an uneasy truce. Most times, I do my thing, and they do their thing. I say that to them often when they flare: *You do your thing and I'll do mine*. But one thing I've come to understand is that the best weapon I've had in dealing with this isn't medication, or meditation, or therapy, but writing.

When I haven't written for a while, any (or all) of these neuroses grow to prominence. It's writing that gives me a vehicle to work out what's going on in my head, and gives me a chance to express myself, thus performing something of an exorcism of these neuroses from myself.

It's a delicate balance, though, because too much writing drains me, and leaves me flat and apathetic, as if I've not only vented and exorcised myself, but also drained myself of the reserves I require to function.

I mention this as a cautionary tale for anybody who will write as a means of self-maintenance.

As with everything in life, you have to find your balance.

An Exercise

Try this: pick a difficult time in your life – a break-up, for example.

And spend five minutes just thinking about how it made you feel.

Then spend five minutes writing about how it made you feel.

Then, after you've read this entire piece, try writing about it again.

Direction

Our thoughts are usually chaotic. They scramble from one, to another, to another, and then back around again. This occurs whether you have a neurotic personality or not. We're all victims of hectic lives, and trying to manage too much in what little time we have.

If you've ever tried to meditate, or simply to sit down, relax, and have five minutes of down time, you'll probably have experienced the way your thoughts will jump around – even if you make a conscious effort to point them in the one direction.

Writing offers a focus – a direction that you take. But it also offers you a freedom. If you were talking to a friend, or counsellor, you might refrain from expressing yourself with complete, uninhibited openness, for fear of the way you'll be judged. And people *do* judge. Think about when somebody's told you something shocking, and you've automatically made some judgement of them. This is just a reality of the way we're brought up. Judgement is imprinted on us as an automatic function of our everyday lives. Our parents judge us by what we do, how we look, and what we want to do. Contemporary life ingrains this in us more than ever where reality shows require we vote people off based on judgement. So it's no surprise we do it with others.

Trying to think things through might give you the freedom to express yourself, but again, thinking can lack direction, and continuity. Sometimes, this might be the mind's own way of protecting you from dealing with painful thoughts. Other times, you get mired in an emotive response.

But when you write, it's you, the page, and whatever you want to say.

But What Do You Want to Say?

If you went to a bookstore, you'd find two sorts of autobiographies out there: tell-all, and (what I call) a press-kit.

Lots of celebrities have press-kit autobiographies out there, books which will detail their life circumstantially, and even talk about how they felt at times, but the books only exist to advertise them – and usually in a positive light. You might learn something about the events of these people's lives, but not really *what* motivates them, *why* it motivates them, and *how* they feel.

A good example of a tell-all autobiography is Andre Agassi's *Open*. Agassi, a former champion tennis player, talks openly about how his father drove him to play tennis from an early age, drove him at all costs, and the crippling fear that rode Agassi through the game, and how it shaped his life.

When I worked as an editor, I read lots of people who'd wanted to tell their life story, but in the end, unwittingly wrote themselves a press-kit. They had lots of interesting things happen, but instead of exploring the way these events made them feel and shaped them, they only reported the events circumstantially, and then stuck on a label that was meant to represent their state emotionally.

For example:

> My father's death left me distraught. I was shattered, and just wasn't sure how I could go on.

Tell me, what exactly is 'distraught'? I'm sure we all know the dictionary meaning of the word, but that's imposing an established definition to reflect an experience which to you *is* unique. Similarly with 'shattered'.

As for 'wasn't sure how I could go on', this is a phrase that's cliché. Clichéd phrases are to be avoided at all costs. They no longer hold real meaning, and simply offer an order of words that constructs a phrase that gives you a convenient yet powerless descriptor, e.g. 'When my partner left me, it broke my heart.' What's a broken heart? How does that feel? What does it really mean?

This is the important thing: you need to reach into yourself, past those protective mechanisms that don't want you facing pain, that try to detour with labels that are convenient, and give expression to how you truly feel.

It will probably hurt, but that's good. Nothing difficult comes easy. If you break a leg, it doesn't heal painlessly. If you're training for a marathon, the training isn't effortless. And if you need to deal with issues, it's not going to be easy.

This is something I've learned myself as a writer. Years ago, I wrote a memoir about dealing with my various neuroses, and commended myself (at the time) having the courage to express myself, and admit what I was experiencing.

That was, in part, true, but it was only years later that I realised I hadn't actually gone very deep into expressing myself – I'd used all the right words and reported everything, but hadn't always admitted my innermost fears, my vulnerabilities, and confronted my own frailties.

When I rewrote the memoir years later, that remained at the forefront of my mind:

Be honest.
Go deep.
Withhold nothing.

Looking back at our original example, imagine it revised as this:

> My father's death opened a gaping chasm in me, a disappointment that I'd never been able to prove myself to him, or show him that I'd made something of myself, that he could be proud of me, and that he could go into the afterlife at least comfortable in the knowledge I'd finally learned to take care of myself.

From those two example passages, which is the more powerful?

Which tells you the most about the way the author feels?

Which would you want to read more of?

Feelings

We deal with issues intellectually, emotionally, physically, and spiritually.

I'm sure all manner of professionals could break it down for you scientifically, but that's how easily I see it – heart (emotion), mind (intellect), body (physical), and soul (spiritual).

When we express ourselves in writing, we need to make sure we attend to each of these facets. Some might be more prominent than others at any given time, but they're all affected.

Think of a time you might have been panicked. You might've experienced:

- shortness of breath, tremors, tightness in your chest (physical)

- distress, flightiness, that you wanted to cry (emotion)
- thoughts that became overly protective of yourself, like you wanted to flee (mind), and
- a despair that you couldn't get through this, that your life had lost meaning (spiritual).

So when you write, question how each of these areas were affected, and express exactly how those areas were affected.

Journals

Journals are a great forum, and they provide any number of avenues. You could write about an event, and portray how it affected you. Or you could vent, and express how something makes you feel. You could address somebody who's wronged you, writing as if you were going to send them a letter. Or, if you're of a more poetic nature, you may write a poem.

This is writing. There's no limit to what you can actually do.

Journals also help us make sense of what's going on inside our heads – stuff that hasn't been articulated. Our writing can give it a shape and form that our mind hasn't (or at least not consciously). This 'sense' mightn't happen immediately. Sometimes, it might be a lengthy process as we unravel on the page, the way a picture takes shape as you put a jigsaw together.

But by providing it an avenue to expression, we let our minds work out exactly how they feel about something on every level.

Through a period of 2010, as I went through a serious bout of my depression (brought on by other at-the-time-undiagnosed health issues), I kept journals in which I wrote letters to people who I felt had wronged me, explored how I was feeling to put it in context and to see how it could be addressed, and also wrote about things I was thankful for in my life. With the latter, it was useful for me to see that life wasn't all bad.

These simple exercises buoyed me at a time I was despondent and unsure about myself, and about what was going on, as well as helped me to put in context what I was feeling and how it was affecting me.

Memoir / Autobiography

Whereas journaling may address specific issues, and may do so in a completely free form, writing memoir (about a period of our lives) or autobiography (writing about all of our life) offers a structure: the arc is our own life.

The goal in writing memoir or autobiography is to think about where your story begins, where it ends, and the journey we undertake – and the journey itself is pivotal. Life is a learning experience. Each day, we try to better ourselves in some way, try to grow in some form. This is the question that's the foundation of what we're writing: *how have we changed during this journey?*

It's little use writing a story where we begin and end at the same point in life, unless our point is to show how we've resisted change.

Agassi's *Open* shows how Agassi begins as

insecure and dominated (by his father), details how he stumbles often, but he learns and grows as a person, until he becomes a mature, responsible, rounded family man with a social conscience.

With my own memoir, and a blog I wrote that covered the decades of my neurosis, I always knew my arc would begin with a kid experiencing things he simply didn't understand (e.g. panic, anxiety, OCD, depression), and which he allowed to dominate him and box him into a corner, dealing with issues symptomatically rather than looking at the cause, and finally reconciling where I'd come to in life, and how any wisdom I'd gain simply through time and experience could be applied to management of my issues (and, thus, my life). It mightn't be some rousing triumph against impossible odds, but it shows how I've grown, how I've changed, and how I'm in a much more comfortable place nowadays than I was twenty years ago, ten years ago, or even just last year.

So if you want to write memoir or autobiography, ask yourself what's the journey you undertake?

Blogging

Blogging allows you the opportunity to share your story with the greater public through serialisation, or episodic instalments. For some, this might seem an opportunity for fame and aggrandisement, but that motivation will only eschew the exploration and interpretation of what you're feeling, like you were sharing your story on some outrageous tabloid talk show. That's not what you want. You want to be true to yourself. You *need* to be true to yourself.

The other power of blogging – besides the potential for catharsis – is that it can help you get in touch with people who are experiencing something similar, or even help you create a community. It's always useful to touch others, and know you're not alone.

As with memoir/autobiography, if you blog you should consider the arc of your story – where does it go and where will it finish? What's the purpose of each blog? To tell part of your story? To deliver a message piecemeal? To educate? There're no limitations, but it's important to keep in mind the purpose behind why you'd want to blog.

My own blog, *The Other Me*, shares a lifetime of neurosis. People have messaged me privately to commend me for having the strength to share, and also to express that they've learned stuff through reading my blog which has helped put their own experiences in context.

That's gratifying to me – I wish when I was nineteen or twenty somebody sat me down and talked me through the anxiety and depression I was going through and help put it in context, instead of what did happen (which was to let it explode out of control because I couldn't make sense of it). If just one person can be helped through reading my story, then (for me) it's worthwhile.

So if you intend to blog, think about *why* you want to blog.

In Fiction

People think fiction is just making stuff up.

But, often, fiction is also a writer's attempt to reinterpret how they're feeling. Some authors will fictionalise a time in their lives, so that their story is just a thinly-veiled recreation of something that happened to them. Others will use different facets of their story – a character might deal with an issue that the author themselves is dealing with, or there might be a subplot that reflects something the author is going through. On occasion, this reinterpretation might happen entirely unconsciously. An author might decide to write a story completely unrelated to their life, and yet some component unintentionally becomes an interpretation of something they are experiencing.

This can happen regardless of what we're writing about. Our stories don't have to be a contemporary microcosm of our own lives, as well as our reality, to reflect what's going on inside us. It can happen through any genre. You might write a fantasy, with sorcerers and dragons and magic kingdoms. Doesn't sound like real life at all, does it? But the antagonist might be a reinterpretation of an ex, or a boss who's mistreated you; the protagonist's mentor might be a parental figure the author's missing; the protagonist's own insecurity about taking on a quest might reflect the author's own insecurity about a life change. These are just examples, but demonstrate how aspects of our lives can find their way into our writing, regardless of what we are writing.

With myself as a writer, often my protagonists

are deeply neurotic or world-shy, are struggling to come to grips with events around them, and often have to reconcile how they'll move forward because, if they don't, their thought processes, their mindset, their neuroses, will get the better of them and either destroy their world, or imprison them in torturous circumstances.

Interestingly, often these protagonists will face issues similar to mine, or which are metaphors for whatever I'm going through. Often, helping them get through whatever they're facing helps me to put in context whatever issue I'm facing at that time, and illuminates a course that I could take.

If nothing else, writing helps me to structure and articulate something that's formless in my head.

Poetry / Verse

I'm not a poet, and whilst I've edited poetry, I've always approached it as I would approach a story – has the author gone deeply enough into a detail, have they truly explored how something made them feel, what did they feel at a given time, etc.?

Because of this, I'm wary to go into the specific benefits of what writing poetry (or verse) offers, but as a form of writing I understand it's simply another form of expression, and one which has its own strengths and virtues, so it's worth mentioning because it has equal validity to every other form of writing I've mentioned.

Be Yourself

Something else that's important when you're writing is to be yourself. You might prefer to sound like Hemingway or write like Plath, but Hemingway and Plath became Hemingway and Plath by *being* Hemingway and Plath.

You should write by being who *you* are.

This is the best way of being true to yourself.

So write freely.

Let it pour from you.

Don't worry about grammar or punctuation or phrasing at this stage.

Don't consult Thesauruses.

Don't try to sound lofty, because you think it adds weight to your writing.

Don't try to moralise.

If you read my early writing, it often had a grand tone, because I wanted to sound older and wiser than my years, and I thought being formal and using big words would help me do that. But as the years have gone on, I've pared it back, until my prose is generally simple, and in doing that, I feel like I'm now being authentic.

Just be who you are, as that's the best way of getting in touch with expressing yourself.

When Writing ...

... always keep in mind the following guidelines:

3. **Be Yourself**: You will write at your best, and at your truest, when you write as yourself.
4. **Go Deeper**: Whenever you've recounted an event, asked yourself if you've gone as deeply into it as you can, or whether you've offered only a cosmetic account.

5. **Cover the Intellectual, Emotional, Physical, and Spiritual Aspects:** You don't have to cover all these simultaneously. In all likelihood, at any given time one or two components will be prevalent, whilst the remainders will fade into the background. But ask yourself, how any and all of these things felt.

I don't have all the answers. I probably don't even have *some* of the answers. But I know how writing has helped keep me balanced over the years, allowing me to interpret and explore my feelings, sometimes directly (through memoir and blogging), sometimes abstractedly (through fiction).

It's a medium without boundaries – not something that many mediums can boast. You're only limited by your own willingness to express yourself, and your wherewithal to delve into your own thoughts, feelings, and inner being.

Whatever form your writing takes, it can help you make sense of issues within yourself that you don't fully understand, as well as the world around you.

Try it and see how you go.

Biographies

Samantha Jansen is on a mission to inspire and motivate individuals who want and believe they deserve more than settling for an average life. She strongly believes you can have anything you want, if you believe in yourself. Samantha grew up in Sri Lanka and came to Australia when she was eighteen, and immediately experienced rejection and hardship within the first twelve months.

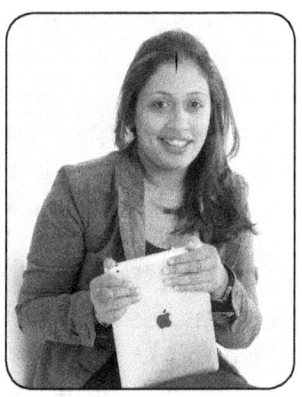

'Every time someone hurt my feelings or challenged me,' she says, 'something within me grew and I knew I was eventually going to prove them wrong. I have used that energy to drive me to achieve my goals and build my ideal lifestyle.'

Samantha worked in a finance company for nine years before starting her own business in 2012. She knows and understands what it is like to think from an employee's headspace. Since starting her business she has created a space for individuals to have an attitude of 'LIVE Life on MY Terms'.

She primarily works with small business owners, but also with individuals considering starting a business, and educates and supports them as they transition and make a change in their life to uncover success while building their ideal lifestyle.

Samantha is an Entrepreneur, a Mentor, a Speaker and Mum to Sierra and Savinesh. She can be contacted by visiting her website, which is www.platform4success.com.

Anthony Kilner is a Psychic Medium, Author, Educational Facilitator, Mentor, Energy Worker, Freelance Photo Journalist, Speaker and Musician. He is also qualified in Trance Healing, Massage and is a Reiki and Seichim Master.

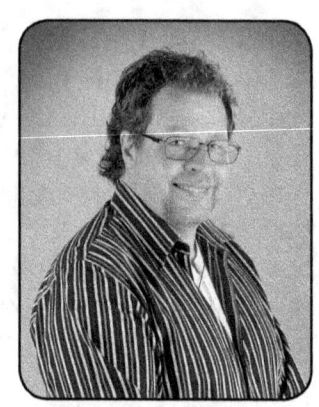

Having studied Vibrational healing in India and Australia, Anthony has come to respect it as a powerful tool to promote ongoing wellbeing as it works on the entire physical body, encouraging self-healing.

After actively working with Spirit for over ten years as a Psychic Medium at various locations, Anthony has now created a beautiful working and teaching environment in Research Victoria where he operates his business – Bridging Realms. Anthony is passionate about assisting people with a holistic approach to living and working and how to find the right work/life balance.

In 2013 he started his newest business, The Spiritual Coach, and also wrote his first book, *Secret Spiritual Business – Unlocking the Power to Holistic Success*, where he shares a plethora of knowledge and personal experiences on how to achieve success while doing what you love and working from home.

Being a passionate musician who understands the healing effects of sound on the body Anthony is also founding member of Divine Light Orchestra

(DLO). DLO's music has been described as a 'celebration of sound' utilising an amazing array of tribal and contemporary instruments.

Dr Galen Dean Loven has always been a personal coach. With many of his clients being business owners, his focus was on integrating personal development with the demands of management. As self-development continued, the depth and quality of his work changed.

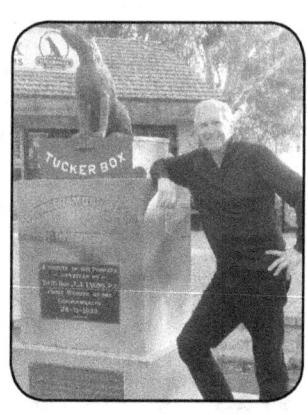

A major evolution occurred twenty years ago when Galen completed his benchmark studies on the relationship of morals and ethics to corporate profit and competitiveness. That statistically accurate proof of a direct relationship launched his journey into discovering ways to balance the heart with the mind. The road was hard as Galen was neither easy on himself, nor able to find 'magic buttons' or shortcuts.

He was blessed with the aid, teaching and support of many beautiful souls and spirits, many of whom experience similar challenges of balancing spirit, heart and mind. Coming to Australia more than three years ago to teach this balance to spiritual professionals and healers, he found a 'home' and VIVA Community Networks Worldwide was born.

This company is a beautiful partnership of

like-minded individuals who think outside the box: VIVA Global, a new company about to become publicly listed on the Budapest Stock Exchange. VIVA Global is the ultimate expression of doing business with heart – making money while making a positive difference to the lives and futures of children throughout the world. A company built on the value of sharing.

More on VIVA Global may be found at www.vcnww.com or contact pam.fallon@vcnww.com

Galen Loven may be contacted at gdl@morals.net. https://galenlovenauthor.wordpress.com/ https://www.facebook.com/theweavesaga

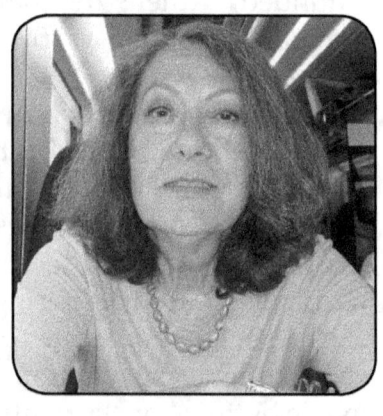

Isolde Martin was born in Germany on the Danube and close to the Austrian border.

She spent her childhood close to Munich. Later, she moved with her family to Munich where she studied, worked, and enjoyed her youth. In 1971, she left for Sydney, Australia, where she spent a year. In 1972, she moved to the USA to study psychology. In 1978, she graduated with a Bachelors degree in Psychology from the George Washington University in Washington, DC. She completed her Masters in Behavioral Sciences in 1981 at the University of Houston, Texas. The next move brought her to California where she took her internship specialising in Art Psychotherapy.

All in all she has lived and worked in six foreign countries, and learned about foreign cultures. She spent over thirty years as an expatriate. Her experiences of life as an expat, and the problems and pleasures coming with it, have been detailed in her autobiography, *Far Away from the Brewery*. Originally written in English, the book has now been published in German.

Isolde now lives again in the Munich area. From there she has published a book, *Notes from the 48th North*, which reflects her ways and mental problems of repatriating in short anecdotes, sometimes poetic, sometimes streams of consciousness, always entertaining.

Mary Jo Mc Veigh BSSC (Hons) MSW is the founder and director of Cara House and CEO of CaraCare, located in Sydney, Australia. She completed her Honours degree in social science in 1983 and worked in her community of North Belfast before returning to university and completing a Master's Degree in Social Work in 1986. She is a trained trauma therapist and an accredited mental health social worker.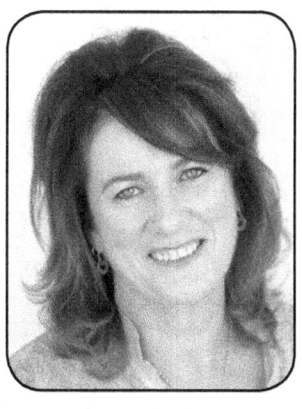

She is acknowledged in her field as an expert in child protection, trauma therapy and leadership coaching. Her expertise has been sought on advisory panels such as the NSW Domestic Violence reforms and the Royal Commission into institutional abuse.

Mary Jo has published an innovative and beautiful resource for resilience building in children and young people. In addition she has written two books: *Discovering Audacious Love*, about her development as a social worker was published in 2012, and *Without Question* in 2015.

Mary Jo has been interviewed in the media in Ireland and Australia about her work and life, featuring in magazine and newspaper print, and appeared on Irish Television and SBS TV as part of an expert panel. She has also been interviewed on radio by the BBC, Ulster radio, 2UE and ABC Radio on *Conversations* with Richard Fidler. She was Canada Bay City Council Woman of the Year in 2010.

She has developed a series of creative leadership courses and has been engaged to run them for the NSW Health Department, Department of Family and Community Services, and Non-Government organisations and leadership conferences.

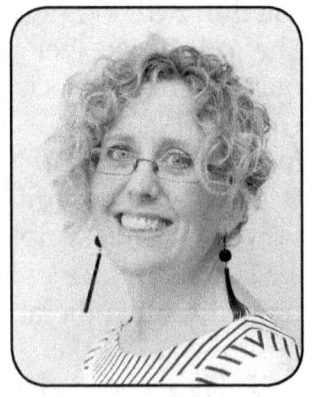

The mother of four children, **Debbie Rossi** was a victim of childhood bullying. As an adult, she felt unable to deal with the emotional scars that the bullying left behind. These feelings were exacerbated when her first daughter started school. Through Debbie's journey to learn Kinesiology, she has been able to break down these internal barriers and thoughts that were preventing her from being confident and happy within herself. Debbie discovered that many of her Kinesiology clients were also going through similar issues of unresolved childhood emotional trauma.

Debbie's book, *Beyond the Schoolyard*, focuses on learning to forgive and let go of past hurts allows healing and growth in the present and future. She teaches that self-love and self-care are the stepping-stones on the path to a more positive and healthy life. Learning to communicate our needs and wants clearly and to care for ourselves allows you to heal and move beyond the hurts of the past.

With a Diploma in Kinesiology, Debbie has been practising Kinesiology for five years. She is also qualified as a Counselling Kinesiology Practitioner. She has a BrainGym 101 and LEAP 1 qualification and is qualified in Flower Essences, specialising in Australian Bush Flower Essences. Debbie is a registered Specialist Kinesiology Practitioner with the Australian Kinesiology Association (AKA).

Dr Talia Steed is a medically-trained Counsellor, Writer and Mental Health advocate. Her professional and personal experiences have shaped her holistic and integrative framework to psychological issues that consider wellbeing from a Body, Mind and Spirit perspective.

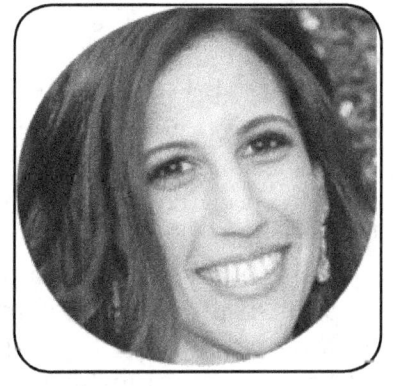

Specialising in women's and children's mental health, Dr Talia has a collaborative and flexible approach that focuses on empowering and assisting her clients uncover their own inner voice, to guide them on their life's path. Dr Talia also values preventative strategies such as yoga and mindfulness meditation for fostering mental wellbeing and creating a rich and meaningful life.

www.drtaliasteedcounsellor.com.au

Blaise van Hecke is co-owner and Publisher at Busybird Publishing. She is also a writer, writing mentor, photographer and artist.

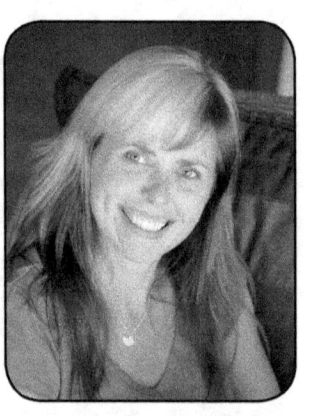

She has been published in the short story anthology, *Mud Puddles* (May 08), *Blue Crow Magazine,* [untitled] issue two, came second in the bi-annual short story competition with the Society of Women Writers of Victoria 2007, for her story 'The Eleventh Summer'; and is the author of *The Book Book: 12 steps to successful publishing,* as well as *Who is a Cheeky Monkey?*. Her photographs have been used for book covers, CD covers and promotional literature.

Blaise enjoys writing and travelling and hopes to publish a book that combines both. She runs various workshops for Busybird about writing, editing, and publishing, and is popularly in demand for talks about publishing in general.

What Blaise loves most is nurturing an author through the self-publishing process, and the look on their face when they finally have their book in their hands.

Find out more about Blaise and her musings about books at www.thebookchick.com.au.

Sara Van Hecke is a clinical psychologist who works with individuals who are struggling with issues including anxiety, depression, parenting and grief. She has extensive experience working with couples and is known for her warm and direct approach. She also has a strong interest in complementary health, particularly in relation to cancer. Her work with women around dealing with breast cancer stems from her own journey with breast cancer.

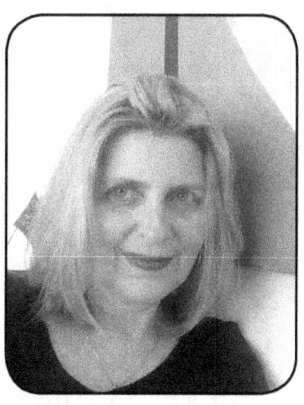

She is the mother of three adult children and has been happily co-habitating with her partner for almost thirty years.

Les Zigomanis is a Melbourne writer who's had stories and articles published in various print and digital journals, had screenplays optioned, and written novels. Some of his short stories and his blogs (including *The Other Me*) can be found at www.leszig.com.

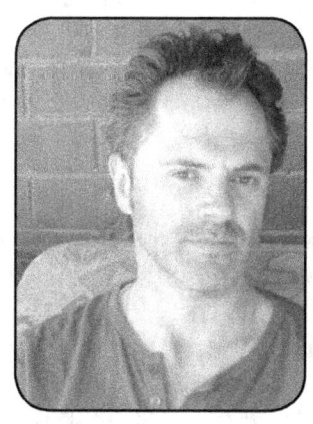

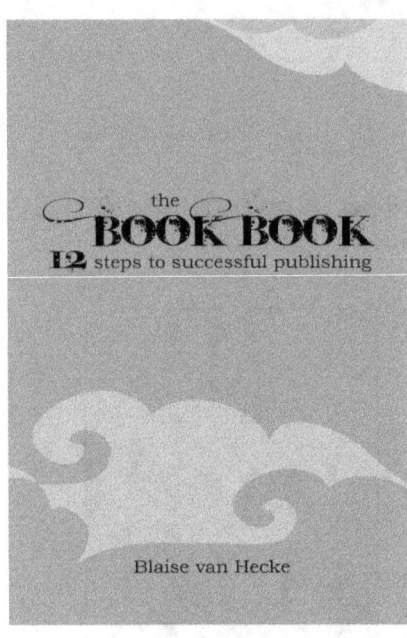

Title: The Book Book
Price: $18.00
Publication Date:
   7 February 2014
Format: Paperback (181x111mm, 148 pages)
ISBN: 978 0 992 4325 0 8
Category: Nonfiction

The Easy Publishing Series is perfect for anybody with an interest in writing, or who's a writer and wondering where to go next.

The Book Book will talk you through the writing and publishing process, providing invaluable tips and insider knowledge into the publishing industry, as well as the inspiration to get started and to keep writing to the end.

The Launch Book will guide you through setting up a book launch, using a simple guide and fun illustrations which'll ensure you celebrate your book's arrival into the world!

If you're a writer and want to publish, or want to look your book, make sure you check out *The Easy Publishing Series*.

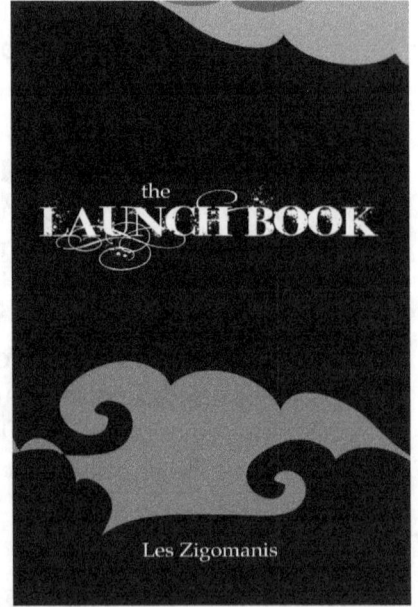

Title: *The Launch Book*
Price: $18.00
Publication Date:
   22 April 2015
Format: Paperback (181x111mm, 70 pages)
ISBN: 978 0 992 5226 0 5
Category: Nonfiction

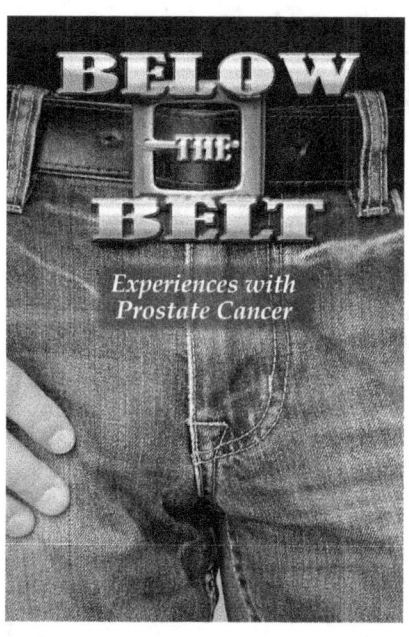

Title: *Below the Belt: Experiences with Prostate Cancer*
Price: $25.00
Publication Date: 21 February 2015
Format: Paperback (153x234mm, 205 pages)
ISBN: 978 0 992 5547 3 6
Category: Nonfiction

Our anthologies on cancer – real people sharing their experiences about what they went through, stories that are honest, heartfelt, and raw.

There's a strength which comes from sharing. In reaching out and touching others, we build communities of knowledge and assurance, we let each other know that we are not alone.

A portion of proceeds from *Journey* will go to BreaCan and WHOW (Women Helping Other Women), while $5.00 from every *Below the Belt* sold will go to the Prostate Cancer Foundation.

Title: *Journey: Experiences with Breast Cancer*
Price: $32.00
Publication Date: 20 February 2012
Format: Paperback (150x230mm, 326 pages)
ISBN: 978 0 987 1538 0 7
Category: Nonfiction

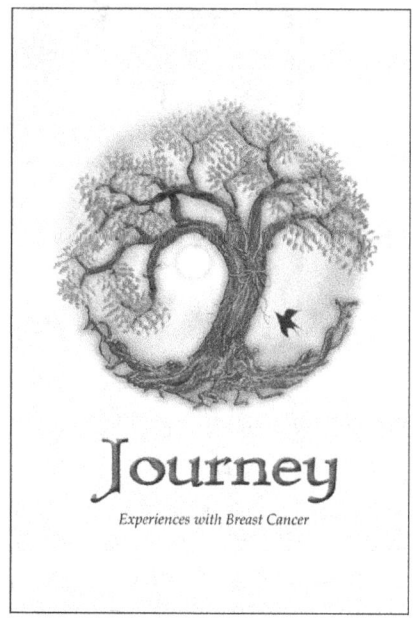

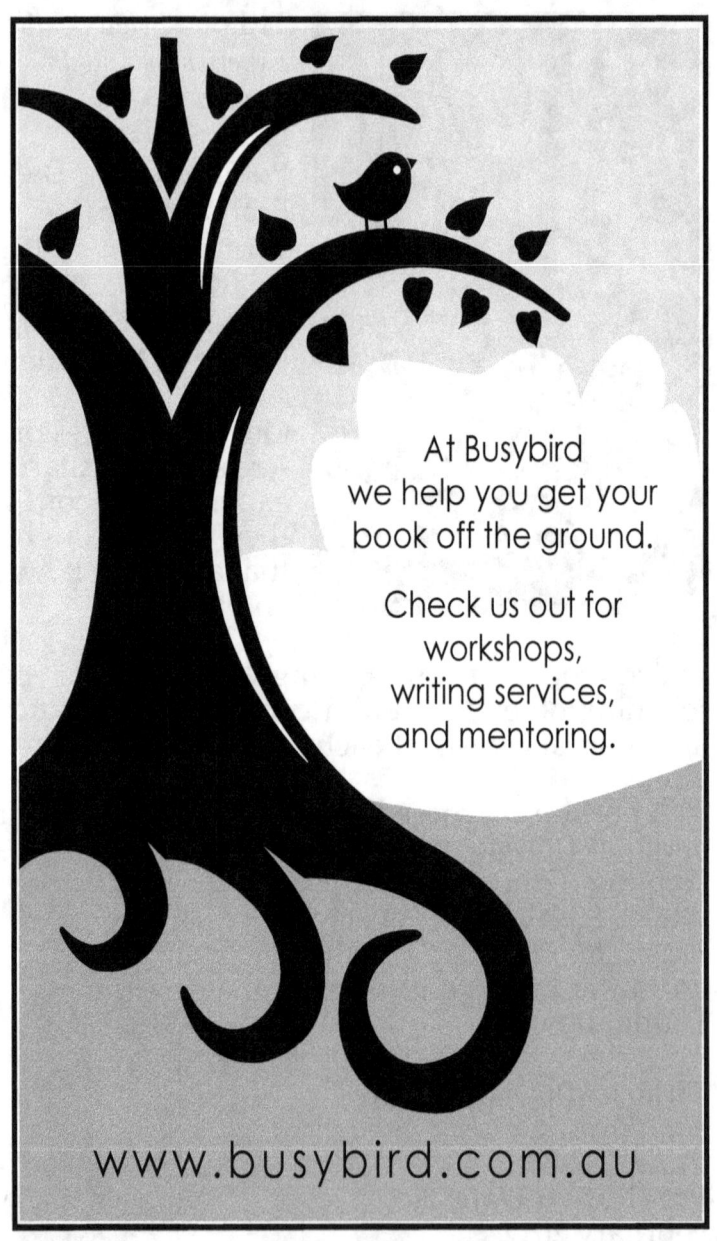

Busybird Publishing is a small, boutique publisher based in the heart of Montmorency, Victoria.

We produce our own range of books, as well as help authors get their stories out into the world.

www.ingramcontent.com/pod-product-compliance
Lightning Source LLC
Chambersburg PA
CBHW071617080526
44588CB00010B/1170